Case-Based Haematology

Professor Shaun McCann MB, FRCPI, FRCPath, FRCPEdin

Professor of Haematology, St James' Hospital Dublin, University of Dublin, Trinity College, Ireland

Professor Robin Foà MD

Professor of Haematology, University 'La Sapienza', Rome, Italy

Professor Owen Smith MA, MB, FRCPI, FRCPEdin, FRCPCH, FRCPath

Consultant Paediatric Haematologist, Our Lady's Hospital for Sick Children and Professor of Haematology, University of Dublin, Trinity College, Ireland

Dr Eibhlin Conneally MB, PhD, MRCPI, FRCPath

Consultant Haematologist & Lecturer in Haematology at the University of Dublin, Trinity College, Ireland

Blackwell
Publishing

© 2005 S. McCann, R. Foà, O. Smith and E. Conneally
Published by Blackwell Publishing Ltd
Blackwell Publishing, Inc., 350 Main Street, Malden, Massachusetts 02148–5020, USA
Blackwell Publishing Ltd, 9600 Garsington Road, Oxford OX4 2DQ, UK
Blackwell Publishing Asia Pty Ltd, 550 Swanston Street, Carlton, Victoria 3053, Australia

The right of the Author to be identified as the Author of this Work has been asserted in accordance with the Copyright, Designs and Patents Act 1988.

First published 2005

Library of Congress Cataloging in Publication Data

Case-based haematology / Shaun McCann ... [et al.].
    p. ; cm.
  ISBN 1-4051-1321-9
  1. Blood--Diseases--Case studies. 2. Hematology--Case studies.
 I. McCann, Shaun R.
  [DNLM: 1. Hematologic Diseases. 2. Case Reports.   WH 120
C337 2004]
 RC636.C37 2004
 616.1'5--dc22

 2004016478

ISBN 1-4051-1321-9

A catalogue record for this title is available from the British Library

Set in 9.5/12 pt Minion by Sparks, Oxford – www.sparks.co.uk
Printed and bound in India by Replika Press PVT Ltd

Commissioning Editor: Vicki Noyes
Development Editor: Geraldine Jeffers
Editorial Assistant: Nic Ulyatt
Production Controller: Kate Charman

For further information on Blackwell Publishing, visit our website:
http://www.blackwellpublishing.com

The publisher's policy is to use permanent paper from mills that operate a sustainable forestry policy, and which has been manufactured from pulp processed using acid-free and elementary chlorine-free practices. Furthermore, the publisher ensures that the text paper and cover board used have met acceptable environmental accreditation standards.

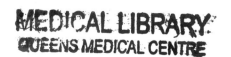

Contents

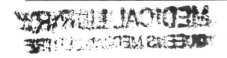

Preface

I hope you enjoy reading this book because I certainly enjoyed writing it! Yes, there are plenty of well-written textbooks on haematology, although most of them are aimed at postgraduates. This book attempts to reconstruct problems as they present in real life in the clinic. There are no long lists of causes of diseases, but there is an attempt to help you to use and develop your thought processes and your powers of logic and deduction. In most hospitals harassed junior staff order countless tests daily, with little knowledge of the reason for the request (except to have the answer for the 'boss' should he/she ask for it on a ward round) and even less ability to interpret the result and to take appropriate action. This book will, I hope, help you to develop a skill in ordering appropriate and meaningful investigations and interpret the results in a way which will help in the management of the clinical problem.

S. McCann, 2004

Acknowledgements

I would like to acknowledge the contributions of my colleagues in St James's Hospital, E.C. and O.S., and R.F. from Rome. I would also like to thank all other colleagues for their help, especially Dr Ronan McDermott in the department of Diagnostic Radiology, Professor D.S. O'Briain, Histopathologist, Professor D.G. Weir, Dr Corrina McMahon and Mr David O'Brien. Drs Clodagh Ryan and Patrick Hayden were immensely helpful with proof reading and made many useful suggestions. Ciara McLoughlin, a final year medical student, helped me in a time of need and very special thanks are due to 5th year medical student Leong Sum for his tremendous typing skills, good humour and incisive comments. Without his help this book might not have seen the light of day! I would like to thank Professor Terry Lappin and James Cogan for illustrations and to all the patients who gave permission for their photographs to be used. Finally, I would like to thank Geraldine Jeffers from Blackwell Publishing who encouraged and supported me throughout this venture.

Glossary

Aetiology cause of disease

Alleles alternative forms of DNA occupying a specific chromosomal locus

Alzheimer's a degenerative disease of the central nervous system leading to dementia and memory loss

Anaemia the occurrence of haemoglobin below the lower limit for the age and gender of the individual

Angina chest pain induced by myocardial ischaemia

Aspirate removing of tissue through suction of a needle

Ataxic an uncoordinated gait (walk)

Autologous stem cell graft the use of stem cells from the individual to reconstitute haemopoiesis following myeloablative chemotherapy

Autosomal recessive a form of inheritance which requires both alleles for manifestation of the effect

Barrier methods condoms/diaphragms

Blind loop syndrome overgrowth of bacteria in a stagnant loop of bowel

Chelation removal of iron from body tissues

Chemotherapy compounds which cause destruction (apoptosis) of malignant cells or infectious agents

Chronic bronchitis productive cough for more than 3 months, recurring

Cirrhosis fibrotic chronic liver damage with regeneration

Coagulopathy deficiency of coagulation proteins leading to bleeding

Coeliac disease a disease caused by allergy to gluten, resulting in villus atrophy and folic acid/iron malabsorption

Complement a complex series of proteins which participate in the immune response

Crohn's disease inflammatory disease, usually of the distal small bowel

CSF cerebrospinal fluid

Cyst a fluid-filled sac

Cytokines low molecular weight proteins which regulate the immune system, haemopoiesis and the inflammatory response

Cytoskeleton protein structure which maintains cell shape

Diverticulum an out-pouching of the mucosa and submucosa, usually of the large bowel

Embolus thrombus (clot) which has moved along a blood vessel

Emphysema destruction of alveoli within the lung

Erythropoiesis synthesis of red cells

Extensor plantar Babinski sign an up-going big toe with fanning of the other toes following stroking of the lateral surface of the foot. Indicates an upper motor neurone lesion

Extramedullary outside the bone marrow

Ferritin a complex of iron and apoferritin. Small amounts are present in plasma and reflect body iron stores

Fibrinogen a soluble protein in plasma that is converted to fibrin (which is insoluble) by thrombin

Gluten a component of wheat

Gout an acute arthritis due to deposition of uric acid crystals in the joints

Granulocytes neutrophils with granules in their cytoplasm

Haemoglobin molecule made up of four globin chains, containing iron and responsible for oxygen transport

Haemolysate contents of destroyed red cells

Haemopoietic relating to the synthesis of the elements of the blood

Haemopoietic stress increased demand on the bone marrow to produce more cells

Hepatic siderosis deposition of iron in the liver

Hepatosplenomegaly enlargement of the liver and spleen

Hypoxaemic reduced oxygen saturation

Immunoglobulins glycoproteins synthesized by B cells (antibodies)

Ineffective erythropoiesis premature destruction of red cells within the bone marrow

Intrathecal into the CSF

Intrauterine growth retardation failure of foetus to develop normally

Karyotype (cytogenetics) analysis of chromosomes

Kyphosis curvature of the spine secondary to collapse of a vertebral body

Lymphadenopathy enlargement of lymph nodes

Lymphomas malignant transformation of lymphocytes within lymph nodes

Lymphoproliferative disease malignant proliferation of lymphocytes in the blood/marrow/lymph nodes

Malaise a feeling of fatigue

Malaria a disease caused by a parasite, which invades red cells and can cause severe haemolysis

Matrix semisolid medium which supports cellular growth

MCH mean corpuscular haemoglobin (see table of normal values)

MCHC mean corpuscular haemoglobin concentration (see table of normal values)

MCV mean corpuscular volume (see table of normal values)

Mediastinum above and anterior to the heart

Megaloblastic asynchronous development of nucleus and cytoplasm in the bone marrow due to a deficiency of vitamin B_{12} or folic acid

Menarche occurrence of the first menstrual period

Metabolism build-up or breakdown of complex molecules

Metastasis spread of neoplastic cells to a distal site

Moiety a portion of a molecule

Monoclonal immunoglobulin light chain derived from a single lymphocyte/plasma cell

Monocytes white cells with single nucleus and blue/grey cytoplasm, the circulation equivalent of tissue macrophages

Myelin a lipoprotein sheath that surrounds axons in the central nervous system (CNS)

Neonatologist physician who looks after newborns

Neoplasm malignant proliferation

Occult not visible (hidden)

Optic fundi posterior part of the eye where small blood vessels are visible

Osteoporosis demineralization of bone

Paraneoplastic a syndrome occurring in association with malignancy but not a direct result of it

Petechiae pinpoint bleeding into the skin

Phagocytosis engulfment and destruction of foreign material by white cells

Pharyngeal web a membrane occurring in the post-cricoid area of the pharynx in severe iron deficiency leading to development of malignant change

Phlebotomy removal of red cells from the circulation

Plethoric fullness due to increased haemoglobin or blood flow

Pneumothorax collapse of lung due to air in the pleural space

Polychromasia a blue/grey colour of young red cells

Portal hypertension increased blood pressure in the portal circulation, usually due to chronic liver disease

Pre-eclampsia a syndrome in pregnancy characterized by hypertension, proteinuria and oedema

Prophylaxis prevention

Radionucleotide a nucleotide labelled with radioactive material

Radiotherapy treatment of malignant disease by gamma rays or X-rays

Remission inability to detect disease following treatment

Reticulocytes young red cells which are able to synthesize small amounts of haemoglobin for 24–48 hours

Reticuloendothelial a widespread system within the body controlling in part the immune response to infection

Rhesus a blood group

Ribosome cellular structure in which protein synthesize occurs

Sclera the white of the eye

Sickling polymerization of Hb S within red cells

Spina bifida congenital lesion with failure to close the spinal cord associated with folate deficiency *in utero*

Spontaneous abortion loss of foetus not due to external manipulation

Thrombophilia inherited prothrombotic states

Transferrin a plasma protein that transports iron.

Tropical sprue progressive mucosal injury to the small bowel probably caused by infection

Unfixed without the addition of formalin

Units of alcohol 1 unit is equivalent to ½ pint of beer or 1 measure of spirits

Urinalysis microscopic and chemical examination of the urine

Vascular dementia dementia due to reduced blood supply to the brain

Venesection removal of blood from a vein

Normal laboratory values

These values may vary from laboratory to laboratory and country to country, depending on the type of equipment used to carry out the assay and the population being tested. It is extremely important to check the reference values in the laboratory which is carrying out the test for your patient. The values given here have been obtained from the laboratory of St James' Hospital Dublin and are in common use in Europe. Results given in brackets are those commonly used in North America.

	Normal range (female)	Normal range (male)
Haemoglobin	11.5–16.4 g/dl	13.5–18.0 g/dl
Red blood cell count (RBC)	4.0–5.2 × 10^{12}/l (10^6/µl)	4.6–5.7 × 10^{12}/l (10^6/µl)
MCV	83–99 fl (µm^3)	
MCH	26.7–32.5 pg/cell	
MCHC	30.8–34.6 g/dl	
Platelet count	145–450 × 10^9/l (10^3/µl)	
White blood cell count (WBC)	4.0–11.0 × 10^9/l (10^3/µl)	
Neutrophils	2.0–7.5 × 10^9/l (10^3/µl)	
Lymphocytes	1.5–3.5 × 10^9/l (10^3/µl)	
Monocytes	0.2–0.8 × 10^9/l (10^3/µl)	
Eosinophils	0.04–0.40 × 10^9/l (10^3/µl)	
Reticulocytes	20–100 × 10^9/l (0.2–1.5%)	
Erythrocyte sedimentation rate (ESR)	0–15 × mm/hour	0–10 mm/hour
Haptoglobin	0.45–2.05 g/l (30–220 mg/dl)	
Vitamin B$_{12}$	150–1000 ng/l (pg/ml)	
Red cell folate	150–1000 ng/l (pg/ml) of packed red cells	
Serum ferritin	20–300 µg/l (ng/ml)	
Transferrin saturation	<38%	
Erythropoietin (EPO)	6.0–25.0 mIU/ml	
Pulse oximetry: O_2 saturation	>96%	
Red cell mass	20–30 ml/kg	
Plasma volume	40–50 ml/kg	
Total blood volume	60–80 ml/kg	

Continued

	Normal range (female)	Normal range (male)
D-dimers	<500 ng/ml	
Fibrinogen	1.5–4.0g/l	
Prothrombin time (PT)	12.0–15.0 sec	
Activated partial thromboplastin time (APTT)	26.0–35.0 sec	
Bilirubin	0–17 µmol/l (0.3–1.1 mg/dl)	
Direct bilirubin	0–7.0 µmol/l (0–0.3 mg/dl)	
Lactic dehydrogenase (LDH)	230–450 IU/l	
Aspartame amino transferase (AST; also SGOT)	7–40 IU/l	
Alkaline phosphatase	40–120 IU/l	
gamma glutamyl amino transferase (GGT)	10–55 IU/l	
Fasting blood glucose	<7.0 mmol/l (<125 mg/dl)	
Potassium	3.5–5.0 mmol/l	
Calcium	2.30–2.70 mmol/l (8.8–10.8 mg/dl)	
Serum creatinine	50–115 µmol/l (0.5–1.3 mg/dl)	
Uric acid	150–470 µmol/l (3–8 mg/dl)	
Albumin	35–50 g/l (3.5–5.0 g/dl)	
Total protein	60–80 g/l (6.0–8.0 g/dl)	
IgG	6.40–15.22 g/l (700–1450 mg/dl)	
IgA	0.48–3.44 g/l (70–370 mg/dl)	
IgM	0.29–1.86 g/l (30–210 mg/dl)	

A tired woman with iron deficiency

Jenny is a 35-year-old Caucasian woman who works as a secretary. Over the last year she has noticed a decrease in her energy, which has become more marked in the last few months. Normally a very active person, she no longer goes hill walking or plays squash because she is 'too tired' at the end of the day.

She has been living with her partner for 5 years and has never been pregnant. She smokes 10 cigarettes a day and drinks 5 units of alcohol weekly, usually at weekends. Her doctor carried out a blood test.

Q1   What could cause her symptoms?

A She could have respiratory disease as she is a smoker, but there is no history of cough or sputum. Cardiovascular disease could explain some of her symptoms, but she is young with no history of cardiovascular symptoms preceding this episode. She could also be anaemic or depressed as the history is fairly non-specific.

The blood test shows that her haemoglobin is low.

Q2   What type of anaemia is a 35-year-old Caucasian woman likely to have?

A The most likely underlying mechanism is iron deficiency, which is a common cause of anaemia, especially in women of child-bearing age.

Q3   How should her anaemia be assessed clinically?

A A history and physical examination looking for clues as to the cause of her anaemia should be undertaken.

Mild degrees of anaemia are difficult to assess clinically. The palmar creases become pale as anaemia progresses. The conjunctival membranes become pale and the sides of the mouth may become sore. In some patients who do not seek medical attention, the anaemia may become very severe and you may see nail changes (spooning of the nails, koilonychia) or there may be dysphagia due to a pharyngeal web.

Some patients who have chronic and severe anaemia develop a craving for potato chips or other substances (pica).

> **Key point**
> It is common for patients to have no physical signs of anaemia other than some degree of pallor.

Q4 What should be done next?

A A full blood count (Table 1.1) and ask for a blood film (Fig. 1.1).

Table 1.1 Full blood count

	Patient's results	Normal range (female)
Hb	8.0 g/dl	11.5–16.4 g/dl
MCV	62 fl	83–99 fl (μm^3)
MCH	19.0 pg/cell	26.7–32.5 pg/cell
MCHC	30 g/dl	30.8–34.6 g/dl
WBC	5.3×10^9/l	$4.0–11.0 \times 10^9$/l (10^3/μl)
Platelets	550×10^9/l	$140–450 \times 10^9$/l (10^3/μl)

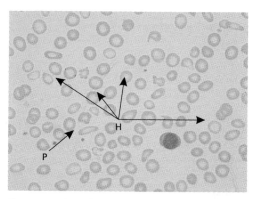

Figure 1.1 Blood film showing red blood cells that are small and pale (H). Pencil shaped cells (P) are also present.

Q5 What do these results indicate?

A Red cells that are small (low MCV) and pale (low MCH) commonly reflect iron deficiency.

> **Key point**
> A deficiency of iron leads to a reduction of haem in the red cells and as a result the rate of synthesis of globin chains is decreased. The platelet count is elevated in patients with iron deficiency even in the absence of blood loss.

Q6 What other reasons could there be that red cells are small and pale?

A Other possibilities are a deficiency in globin chain synthesis (thalassaemia) or the anaemia of chronic disease.

Q7 What reasons would you give, for and against, the aforementioned diagnoses?

A The inherited disorders of haemoglobin synthesis, thalassaemias, are uncommon in Caucasians but are seen in people from the Mediterranean, Middle East and South East Asia. The symptoms and blood findings in patients with thalassaemia will depend on the degree of severity of the genetic defect. People with mild forms of thalassaemia may also suffer from iron deficiency. The anaemia of 'chronic disease' is seen in patients with chronic inflammatory disorders or cancer. It does not seem likely that this patient has cancer or a chronic inflammatory disease.

Q8   What other investigations will help to confirm your suspected diagnosis?

A In most instances measurement of the serum ferritin level will give you an accurate reflection of the iron status. Serum ferritin is low in iron deficiency and is normal in thalassaemia and normal or raised in the anaemia of chronic disease.

> **Key point**
> Normal range for serum ferritin is 20–300 µg/l (ng/ml).

Q9   At what level of serum ferritin would you be prepared to accept iron deficiency as the probable diagnosis?

A A level of <10 µg/l (ng/ml).

Q10   It is likely that Jenny has iron deficiency – what is the next step?

A Take a detailed dietary history and assess iron intake.

In order to try to uncover the underlying cause of her iron deficiency consideration must be given to the way the body handles iron. The daily intake and the daily requirements for iron are almost equal. Therefore, anything which increases iron requirements or causes chronic iron loss, e.g. bleeding, will result in iron deficiency.

> **Key point**
> In healthy adults the majority of dietary iron is not absorbed. However, this can be increased in iron deficiency by 20–30%. Iron is absorbed from the proximal small bowel.

Most body iron is contained in circulating red blood cells. When red blood cells die in the reticuloendothelial system, the iron is re-utilized for the synthesis of haemoglobin. After red blood cell death the iron in the macrophages is transferred to plasma transferrin and then to the maturing red blood cell precursors in the bone marrow, which have transferrin receptors. The amount of iron required on a daily basis to compensate for iron loss due to shedding of enterocytes (the epithelial cells lining the GIT) into the gut and growth requirements is almost identical to iron availability from the diet. Therefore, any excess iron loss is easily converted into iron deficiency anaemia. Menstruating females are thus particularly prone to iron deficiency anaemia.

Q11   What contribution is dietary deficiency likely to make to Jenny's iron deficiency?

A It would be very unlikely that a dietary deficiency of iron would be the sole cause of her anaemia. Jenny has a full time job, a steady relationship and appears well nourished.

Normally, iron is absorbed into the enterocytes via a 'transporter' called DMT-1. The synthesis of DMT-1 reflects the ferritin levels. In iron deficiency, when ferritin levels are low there is less iron in the enterocyte. This leads to an increase in the synthesis of DMT-1, which causes an in-

crease in iron entering the enterocyte. Likewise, the levels of ferritin and transferrin receptor (TfR) are linked. In iron deficiency, ferritin is low and TfR increased. Thus, the synthesis of DMT-1 and TfR respond to physiological needs.

> **Key point**
> Iron deficiency is never a diagnosis on its own. You must always try to find the underlying cause.

A Excessive menstrual blood loss is the most likely cause of iron deficiency in this patient.

Blood loss in excess of 80 ml per month is called menorrhagia. In practice, it is very difficult to assess the menstrual blood loss accurately. Both doctor and patient are likely to overestimate or underestimate the loss. A detailed menstrual history should be taken. Young girls who are at the menarche may bleed excessively before a regular pattern of ovulation is established. Likewise, women who are reaching the menopause commonly have excessive menstrual blood loss.

> **Key point**
> If a patient has a change in the pattern of any symptoms/signs he/she should be referred for investigation.

Q13 What other parts of the physical examination are important in trying to find the cause of iron deficiency?

A A rectal examination with assessment for occult blood in the stool is mandatory.

> **Key point**
> In a post-menopausal female or in a male, blood loss from the gut should be excluded. Peptic ulcer disease, reflux oesophagitis (Fig. 1.2) and cancer of the oesophagus, stomach or large bowel (Fig. 1.3) should be out-ruled by endoscopy. The use of aspirin and non-steroidal anti-inflammatory drugs may cause gastritis and bleeding.

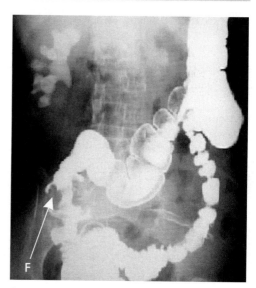

Figure 1.3 A barium enema, showing a filling defect in the caecum (F), due to cancer. As the faeces are liquid in the caecum there may be no change in bowel habit and iron deficiency due to occult blood loss may be the presenting feature. A staghorn calculus is present in the right kidney.

The test for occult blood was negative.

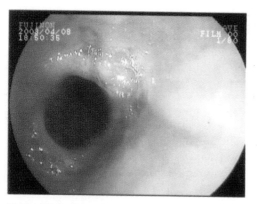

Figure 1.2 Endoscopic examination of the oesophagus showing oesophagitis and bleeding. This may cause retro-sternal (behind the breast bone) pain or may be asymptomatic and present as iron deficiency.

> **Key point**
> Blood loss from the bowel may be intermittent, therefore a single negative test for occult bleeding is not conclusive.

Q14   What other disease mechanisms could lead to iron deficiency?

A Malabsorption due to coeliac disease (Figs 1.4 and 1.5) can present with iron deficiency.

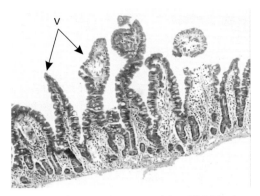

Figure 1.4 The normal pattern of the villi (V) in the small bowel.

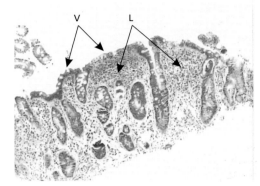

Figure 1.5 Flattened villi (V) and lymphocyte (L) infiltrate present in coeliac disease.

Q15   How can the normal stature, lack of diarrhoea and anaemia be compatible with a diagnosis of coeliac disease?

A Many adults with coeliac disease are of normal stature and have anaemia only.

Q16   If a diagnosis of coeliac disease is suspected, what further tests should be done?

A Tissue transglutaminase antibodies (tTG) in the patient's serum are a reliable index of coeliac disease and, if positive, a duodenal or jejunal biopsy should be carried out to confirm the diagnosis.

A Yes.

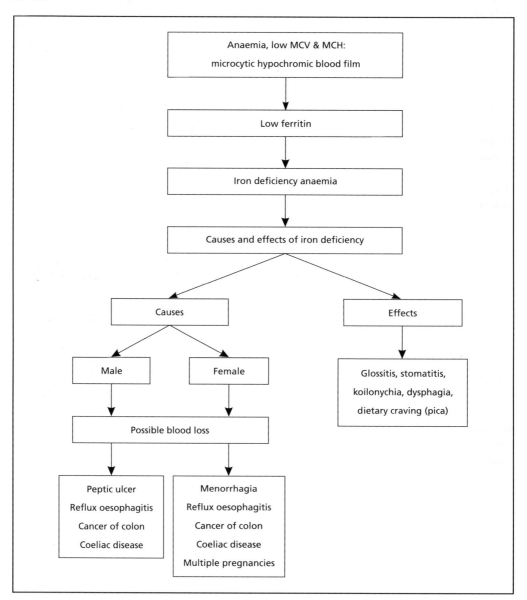

Q18 What are the principles of treatment?

A Treat the underlying disease and give iron replacement.

Q19 How does the method of giving iron (intravenously or intramuscularly) influence the rate of Hb response?

A The blood count will NOT recover more quickly with injections rather than tablets. In the majority of patients iron replacement should be undertaken while the underlying disease is being treated.

Oral iron therapy is almost always successful. Patients should remain on iron therapy for 6 months to ensure adequate replacement of iron stores. In rare circumstances, such as severe iron deficiency of pregnancy, intravenous iron may be used.

> **Key point**
> If the patient does not respond (a rise in Hb of approximately 1g/dl every 3 weeks) reconsider the diagnosis.

OUTCOME

The patient had an upper GIT endoscopy and was found to have reflux oesophagitis and bleeding. This was believed to be the cause of her anaemia. She was advised to stop smoking and restrict her alcohol intake. She was given oral iron replacement for 6 months. She was given a course of proton pump inhibitors and advised to return to her family doctor in 2 months for a blood count. When she went to her family doctor her Hb was 11.5 g/dl and she was advised to take the iron tablets for a further 5 months to replenish her iron stores.

Suggested reading

Centre for Disease Control (1998) Recommendations to prevent and control iron deficiency in the United States. *MMWR*, April 03, 1998/47 (RR-3); 1.36.

Lee, G. Richard (1999) Iron deficiency and iron-deficiency anemia. In: *Wintrobe's Clinical Hematology* (eds G.R. Lee, J. Foerster, J. Lukens, F. Paraskevas, J.P. Greer & G.M. Rodgers), 10th edn, pp. 979–1131. Williams and Wilkins, Baltimore, USA.

Rockey, D.C. (1999) Occult gastrointestinal bleeding. *New England Journal of Medicine*, **341** (1), 38–46.

Hoffbrand, A.V., Pettit, J.E. & Moss, P.A.H. (2001) *Essential Haematology*, 4th edn. Blackwell Science, Oxford. See Chapter 3: Hypochromic anaemias and iron overload.

Frazer, D.M. & Anderson, G.A. (2001) Intestinal iron transport and its regulation. *Hematology*, **6**, 193–203.

A tanned man with diabetes mellitus

Mr Peter Black, a 50-year-old engineer, went to his family doctor complaining of fatigue for at least a year, which was slowly increasing. He said he could only sleep for a few hours and woke early in the morning. He also complained of intermittent pain in the joints of his right hand.

Q1   What are the possible explanations for his complaints?

A Early-morning waking may suggest depression. More information is needed regarding his sleeping pattern and activity levels during the day.

On further questioning, Peter mentioned that he had gone to another doctor, with the same symptoms, 6 months previously. He had been under a lot of pressure at work and the first doctor felt that his symptoms were stress related. He had been prescribed sleeping tablets, which he felt were not helping.

Q2   What further information is needed?

A More information about his joint pain. A history of trauma, swelling or redness of the joints should be sought. One should also enquire about associated symptoms such as weight loss, fevers, night sweats or recent infections.

He revealed that he drank two gin and tonics in the evening and two glasses of wine with his dinner. He is a non-smoker.

On examination Peter is tanned and overweight. His liver is slightly enlarged. His second metacarpophalangeal joint is tender but not red or swollen.

Q3   What else in his history may be contributing to his symptoms and signs?

A His consumption of 28 units of alcohol weekly.

Although alcohol often helps people fall asleep, it also fragments the sleep pattern.

> **Key point**
> Guidelines for sensible drinking suggest that a man should not drink more than 21 units/week (one glass of beer or wine or one spirit measure). Many people who abuse alcohol can continue to function at quite a high level.

A A full blood count (Table 2.1), to see if the fatigue is caused by anaemia; a biochemistry profile and blood glucose (Table 2.2), to find the reason for the enlarged liver.

Table 2.1 Full blood count

	Patient's results	Normal range (male)
Hb	16.5 g/dl	13.5–18.0 g/dl
MCV	100 fl	83–99 fl (μm^3)
WBC	6.0×10^9/l	$4–11.0 \times 10^9$/l (10^3/μl)
Platelets	160×10^9/l	$140–450 \times 10^9$/l (10^3/μl)

The white cell differential was normal.

Table 2.2 Biochemical results

	Patient's results	Normal range
AST (SGOT)	60 IU/l	7–40 IU/l
Alkaline phosphatase	140 IU/l	40–120 IU/l
GGT	80 IU/l	10–55 IU/l
Random blood glucose	13.0 mmol/l	<11.1 mmol/l (<200 mg/dl)

Mr Black returned to the surgery 2 weeks later. He was still fatigued, despite stopping the sleeping tablets and reducing his alcohol intake. He mentioned that he was impotent, which he had been too embarrassed to mention initially.

A The elevated blood glucose suggests diabetes mellitus. His liver blood tests are also slightly abnormal. Although his haemoglobin is normal, his red cells are slightly larger than normal (elevated MCV).

A The reticulocyte count, serum vitamin B_{12} and red cell folate level (Table 2.3).

Table 2.3 Reticulocytes and vitamins

	Patient's results	Normal range
Reticulocyte count	$75 \times 10^9/l$	$50-100 \times 10^9/l$ (0.5–1.5%)
Serum B_{12}	600 ng/l	150–1000 ng/l (pg/ml)
Red cell folate	250 µg/l of packed red cells	150–1000 ng/l (pg/ml)

Q7 How can these results be interpreted?

A Large red cells (high MCV) could be reticulocytes due to haemolysis. The vitamin levels are normal and therefore are not the cause of the high MCV. In liver disease lipid accumulates on the red cell membrane causing a macrocytosis.

Q8 In view of these findings, what other information should be sought from the patient?

A A detailed family history should be obtained because some types of liver disease are familial.

He said his father had diabetes mellitus, but also had many other medical problems and had died from cirrhosis of the liver. He said this always surprised him, as his father was a non-drinker.

Q9 What should be done next?

A He should be re-examined for evidence of complications of diabetes mellitus.

His blood pressure is normal. He has gynaecomastia (enlargement of the breast tissue) (Fig. 2.1). His liver span is 18 cm (normal 12–15 cm) (Fig. 2.2). There is no evidence of a peripheral neuropathy. Retinal examination is normal. Urinalysis shows glucose but no protein.

> **Key point**
> As the blood glucose estimation was carried out on a random sample, Mr Black was advised to have the test repeated when he was fasting (Table 2.4).

Table 2.4 Fasting blood glucose

	Patient's results	Normal range
Fasting blood glucose	9 mmol/l	<7.0 mmol/l (<125 mg/dl)

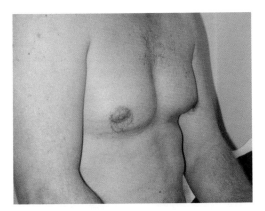

Figure 2.1 Enlargement of the breast tissue in a male, known as gynaecomastia.

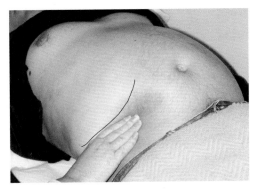

Figure 2.2 Palpation of an enlarged liver. The liver is not normally palpable. In this case, the lower edge is easily felt 3 cm below the costal margin.

Q10 Based on the blood results is a diagnosis possible, and if so what is it?

A Diabetes mellitus, because of the combination of an elevated fasting blood glucose (9.0 mmol/l or greater) and glycosuria. The impotence could be related to a diabetic neuropathy but the gynaecomastia and arthritis are probably not related to the diabetes. The complications of diabetes and the follow-up care and diet should be explained.

He returned in 2 months' time. He had started an exercise programme, modified his diet and lost 5 kg (11.0 pounds). However, he was still complaining of fatigue and a sore hand. The impotence had not improved.

On re-examination, he is pigmented. His liver remains enlarged. He has loss of body hair and the gynaecomastia is more pronounced.

> **Key point**
> He mentions that his cousin was recently diagnosed as having liver problems and was told his iron levels were too high.

Q11 What is the relevance of Mr Black's family history to his diagnosis?

A It is probably very relevant. His cousin has liver disease and was told he had 'too much' iron in his blood. Mr Black's father also had liver disease and diabetes mellitus.

Q12 What connection, if any, can be made between the diabetes mellitus, the liver disease, which appears to be familial, and the clinical findings?

A A genetically inherited disorder in which the body absorbs more iron than is required for daily use is called haemochromatosis.

Because the body has no effective mechanism for excreting iron, other than bleeding, the clinical manifestations of haemochromatosis are much more common in men than women until after the menopause (when monthly blood loss ceases).

A By measuring the serum ferritin and transferrin saturation (Table 2.5).

The serum ferritin concentration is a good measure of body iron stores, but can, however, be non-specifically elevated in inflammatory conditions. The serum transferrin saturation is the most sensitive and cost-effective screening test.

Table 2.5 Iron studies

	Patient's results	Normal range
Transferrin saturation	77%	<38%
Ferritin level	4250 µg/l	20–300 µg/l (mg/ml)

There is no absolute abnormal value, but transferrin saturations of >55–60% in a man or >45–50% in a woman are very suggestive of haemochromatosis.

In 1996, mutations in the *HFE* gene were described and subsequently found in the majority of patients with hereditary haemochromatosis (HH). Two separate mutations have been described; the most common is the C282Y defect where a cysteine residue is replaced by a tyrosine residue. 90% of patients with HH are homozygous for the C282Y mutation. The second defect is H63D where aspartate replaces histidine. These gene mutations can be detected by a DNA-based test.

Mutation analysis showed he was homozygous for C282Y mutation. Figure 2.3 shows DNA, which has been amplified, from normal controls and homozygotes and heterozygotes for the HFE mutant alleles.

Multiplex site-directed mutagenesis PCR plus BbrPI digest for simultaneous detection of the two common hereditary haemochromatosis mutations C282Y and H63D

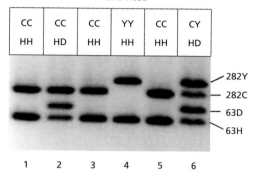

Figure 2.3 PCR (polymerase chain reaction) is used to amplify normal and mutant DNA. Lanes 1, 3 and 5 are normal. Lane 2 is a heterozygote for the H63D mutation. Lane 4 is homozygous for the C282Y mutation (haemochromatosis) and lane 6 is a heterozygote for the two different mutations. Reproduced with kind permission from Caitriona King, National Centre for Medical Genetics, Our Lady's Hospital for Sick Children, Dublin.

Key point

The carrier rate for HH in people of northern European descent is between 10–15%, making it the commonest genetic disorder in this population.

Dietary iron is transported into the enterocyte (cells lining the gut) by the divalent metal transporter DMT_1, among others. The amount of iron absorbed and transported to body stores is regulated by a number of proteins including HFE (the *HFE* gene is on chromosome 6) found in enterocytes and liver cells. The precise mechanism whereby the mutated protein increases iron absorption is unknown but HFE works in conjunction with β2-microglobulin.

Q14 How might the diagnosis of hereditary haemochromatosis (HH) explain Mr Black's symptoms?

A Increased absorption of dietary iron leads to organ dysfunction, especially of the liver, heart, skin and pancreas. This would account for the skin pigmentation, diabetes and abnormal liver blood tests.

Disruption of hypothalamic–pituitary function due to iron deposition leads to hypogonadism, gynaecomastia and impotence.

Arthropathy, due to iron deposition, is a common feature and occurs in 25–50% of patients. The joints of the hands, especially the 2nd and 3rd metacarpophalangeal joints, are usually the first joints involved.

Q15 How should Mr Black be treated?

A Phlebotomy should be performed until his ferritin level falls below 50 µg/l (mg/ml), followed by life-long maintenance phlebotomy.

Mr Black should be referred to a hepatologist to be assessed for evidence of cirrhosis. Once cirrhosis develops, there is >200-fold increased risk of developing liver cancer. Phlebotomy is effective at improving a sense of well-being, normalising the skin pigmentation and liver enzymes. The effect on arthralgia, diabetes and hypogonadism is more variable.

> **Key point**
> Death is most commonly due to cardiac and liver iron overload. If aggressive phlebotomy is initiated before end-organ damage occurs, life expectancy of patients with hereditary haemochromatosis can be normal.

Q16 Mr Black says that he has three teenage children and wonders should they be tested?

A They should be tested because phlebotomy, in affected individuals, will prevent organ damage due to iron excess.

> **Key point**
> The disease is transmitted as an autosomal recessive condition; therefore, homozygotes (individuals with two mutant alleles) may have clinical manifestation of disease. Heterozygotes (individuals with a single mutant allele) are common and usually will not have evidence of disease. In HH, as in other genetic diseases, there is incomplete penetrance, which means that although two people have the same mutation there is marked variability in the level of expression of the disease (Figs 2.4–2.6).

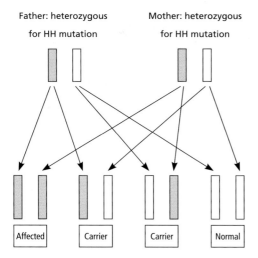

Figure 2.4 The possibilities for the children of a heterozygous mother and a heterozygous father. Blue box designates a mutant allele; white box designates a normal allele.

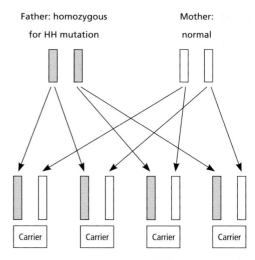

Figure 2.6 The possibilities for children of a homozygous father (haemochromatosis) and a 'normal' mother. Blue box designates a mutant allele; white box designates a normal allele.

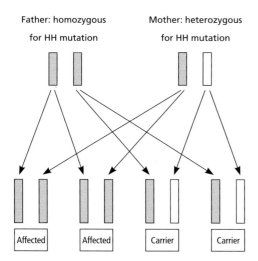

Figure 2.5 The possibilities for children of a homozygous father (haemochromatosis) and a heterozygous mother. Blue box designates a mutant allele; white box designates a normal allele.

A Not practical.

Variable penetrance means that not all patients with the mutations will develop evidence of iron overload. Estimates suggest that it may be as low as 1%. There are also broader issues to bear in mind, such as the use of personal genetic information for the determination of life insurance policies. Up to 40% of individuals at risk of haemochromatosis could be identified by screening of 1st-degree to 3rd-degree relatives of patients with iron overload.

Q18 Can you now construct an algorithm for a patient with pigmented skin and diabetes mellitus?

A Yes.

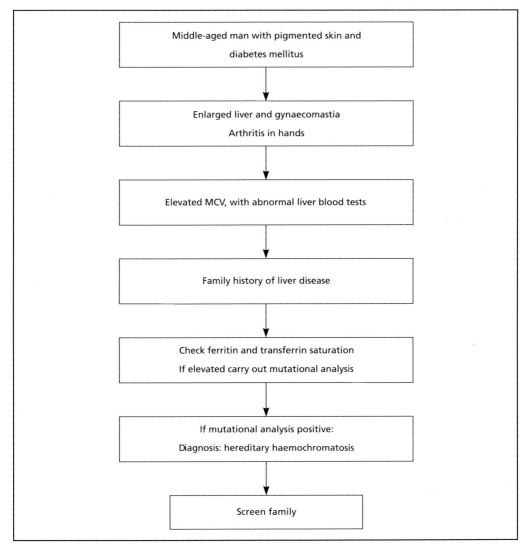

OUTCOME

Mr Black was started on weekly phlebotomy. He will be reviewed every 3 months and more blood removed to keep his ferritin level within the normal range.

His liver blood tests and MCV returned to normal. His blood sugar was controlled by diet. His impotence recovered but his hand remained painful.

Suggested reading

Felitti, V. & Butler, E. (1999) New developments in hereditary hemochromatosis. *American Journal of Medical Science*, **318**, 257–68.

Olynyk, J.K., Cullen, D.J., Aquilla, S., Rossi, E., Summerville, L. & Powell, L.W. (1999) A population-based study of the clinical expression of the hemochromatosis gene. *New England Journal of Medicine*, **341**, 718–24.

Genetic Haemochromatosis. Darwin 2000. British Society for Haematology website.

Beutler, E., Felitti, V.J., Kosiol, J.A., Ho, N.J. & Gelbart, T. (2002) Penetrance of 845G-A (C282Y) HFE in hereditary hemochromatosis mutation in the USA. *Lancet*, **359**, 211–18.

British Committee for Standards in Haematology (2000) Guidelines on diagnosis and therapy. British Society for Haematology website.

Genetic Disorder profile: Hemochromatosis. Gene Gateway-Exploring genes and genetic disorders. Adapted from NIH publication no 02–4621. August 2002.

A cranky lady with jaundice

Brian phoned the doctor's surgery. He said his mother, who was 65 years old, was unwell. She had been deteriorating over a period of 6 months, and recently she was very cranky and her memory had worsened. She seemed short of breath when she came to answer the door and he thought her eyes looked a little yellow.

Q1   What might explain her symptoms?

A Gradual deterioration and irritability could be due to depression. Loss of memory for recent events tends to occur with advancing age. Alzheimer's disease must be considered. Shortness of breath could be cardiac or respiratory in origin. There is nothing in the history to suggest lung disease. Yellow sclera indicates jaundice. Painless jaundice in a woman of her age might suggest carcinoma of the pancreas, haemolysis, or hepatitis.

He was asked to bring his mother to surgery.

Q2   What further information should be sought from the patient?

A A full medical, family and social history. Previous illnesses such as gall bladder disease or jaundice should be enquired about. Shortness of breath in bed at night or on exertion and ankle swelling would suggest heart disease. Previous surgery, especially for cancer, would be very important as she may now have liver metastases. Questions should be asked to assess her degree of memory deficit using the MMSE (Mini Mental State Examination).

She has one sister, aged 70 years, who has 'thyroid problems'. She had a 'fuzzy feeling' in her feet and toes recently. She was a non-smoker and non-drinker. She was normally a placid individual but noticed she was definitely irritable, for the last 6 months. Her husband had remarked that he noticed a slight 'yellowish tinge' to her eyes a few months ago.

Q3   What should be done next?

A A complete physical examination.

She was slightly jaundiced and her skin had a lemon yellow tinge.

Her blood pressure was 130/85 mmHg. Jugular venous pressure (JVP) was raised and there was minimal pitting oedema in both ankles. Deep tendon reflexes in her ankles and knees were absent. The plantar reflex was extensor (Babinski's sign). Appreciation of light touch was poor in both feet and legs. Her walk was slightly ataxic.

Q4 What is the differential diagnosis?

A The neurological findings raise the possibility of diabetes mellitus, but this would not account for her jaundice. An autoimmune disease or a vasculitis causing heart failure, hepatitis and a neuropathy should also be considered. Her sister could have autoimmune thyroid disease. She could have underlying cancer with a paraneoplastic neuropathy, but this would not explain her heart failure.

Q5 What investigations should be done?

A A full blood count (Table 3.1), blood film (Figs 3.1 and 3.2), liver, bone and renal profile (Table 3.2), an ECG and a chest radiograph. The ECG showed a sinus tachycardia and the chest radiograph showed evidence of mild heart failure.

Table 3.1 Full blood count

	Patient's results	Normal range
Hb	7.0 g/dl	11.5–16.4 g/dl
MCV	112 fl	83–99 fl (μm³)
MCH	30 pg/cell	26.7–32.5 pg/cell
MCHC	32 g/dl	30.8–34.6 g/dl
RBC	2.2 × 10¹²/l	4.00–5.20 × 10¹²/l (10⁶/μl)
WBC	2.1 × 10⁹/l	4.0–11.0 × 10⁹/l (10³/μl)
Platelets	98 × 10⁹/l	150–450 × 10⁹/l (10³/μl)

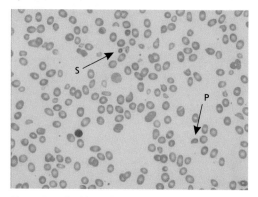

Figure 3.1 The blood film shows anisocytosis (variation in size, S) and poikilocytosis (variation in shape, P).

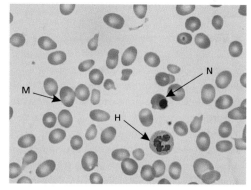

Figure 3.2 A nucleated red blood cell precursor (normoblast, N), a hypersegmented granulocyte (H) and macrocytes (M), larger than normal red cells.

Table 3.2 Biochemical results

	Patient's results	Normal range
Bilirubin	28 μmol/l	0–17 μmol/l (0.3–1.1 mg/dl)
Lactic dehydrogenase (LDH)	>5000 IU/l	230–450 IU/l
Potassium	2.8 mmol/l	3.5–5.0 mmol/l

Q6   **How can the laboratory and clinical findings be linked?**

A The patient is anaemic and jaundiced and the LDH is raised. These findings suggest premature destruction of red cells in the circulation (haemolysis) or in the bone marrow (ineffective erythropoiesis). This degree of anaemia in a patient of this age could cause heart failure, accounting for the oedema and raised JVP. The absence of deep tendon reflexes and the extensor plantar response suggest a combination of upper and lower motor neuron lesions.

Q7   **What blood test might help to clarify if the problem is related to haemolysis or ineffective erythropoiesis?**

A A reticulocyte count (Table 3.3).

Table 3.3 Reticulocyte count

	Patient's result	Normal values
Reticulocyte count	$25 \times 10^9/l$	$50–100 \times 10^9/l$ (0.2–1.5%)

The reticulocyte count is low, suggesting ineffective erythropoiesis. The reticulocyte count reflects the ability of the bone marrow to respond to anaemia. A high reticulocyte count is expected if haemolysis is occurring and a low reticulocyte count would be expected if there is ineffective erythropoiesis. The low white cell and platelet counts also suggest that there is ineffective haemopoiesis.

Q8   **What essential 'building blocks' could become deficient and cause the laboratory and clinical findings?**

A Vitamin B_{12} or folic acid.

Vitamin B_{12} (cobalamin) and folic (pteroylglutamic) acid are both essential for DNA synthesis. A deficiency of either results in abnormal cell production in all body organs. The marrow is a rapidly proliferating organ. Consequently, B_{12} or folic acid deficiency will manifest themselves early in the peripheral blood. Once ingested, dietary vitamin B_{12} is attached to a glycoprotein, intrinsic factor (IF), which is secreted by the gastric parietal cells. The B_{12}–IF complex binds to a receptor in the terminal ileum where B_{12} is absorbed (Fig. 3.3) and transported in the portal circulation, bound to transcobalamin 2 (TC2). The normal diet contains up to 20 µg per day and the daily requirement is 1–2 µg. Therefore, the daily intake greatly exceeds requirements. The vitamin is found in animals only and is not affected by cooking. Body stores of B_{12} (in

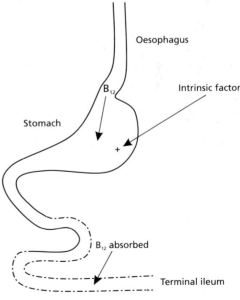

Figure 3.3 The absorption of Vitamin B_{12}.

the liver) should last about 4 years. It is a cofactor for methionine synthase, which methylates homocysteine producing methionine. Methyl-tetrahydrofolate (THF) is the methyl donor in this reaction. Methionine is in turn converted into S-adenosyl methionine, which is involved in most of the methylation reactions in the body, for example the methylation of deoxyribonucle-otides (DNA) and myelin (Fig. 3.4).

Folates consist of a number of compounds derived from pteroylglutamic (folic) acid and are found in most foods including vegetables. They are absorbed through the duodenum and jejunum. An average diet contains about 200 µg, about 50% of which is absorbed. Daily requirements are approximately 100 µg and in sharp contrast to B_{12}, body stores last about 3 months. Folates can be destroyed by cooking.

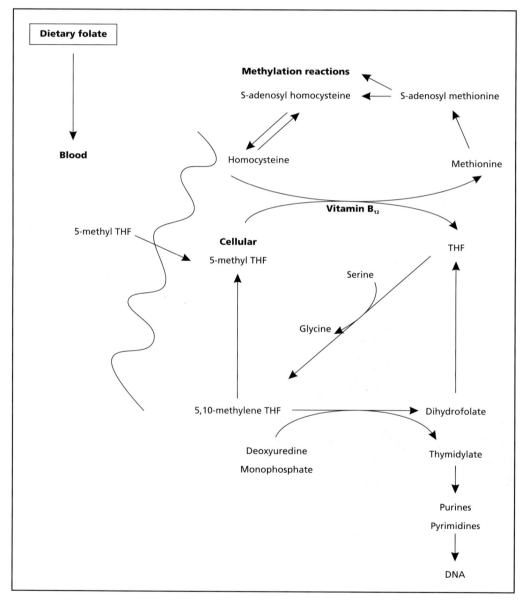

Figure 3.4 The interactions of B_{12} and folate in DNA synthesis.

A Vitamin B$_{12}$ deficiency is most likely because the symptoms are of gradual onset and she has a normal diet, a history of autoimmune disease and neurological damage.

A Measure serum B$_{12}$, red cell folate levels, parietal cell and intrinsic factor (IF) antibodies (Table 3.4). Give her potassium replacement by mouth. Check for other autoantibodies. Start the patient on replacement therapy with oral folate, 5 mg daily, and intramuscular B$_{12}$, 1.0 mg every 3 days for 3 weeks. Check her serum potassium for the first few visits to make sure that the level returns to normal. A bone marrow examination could be carried out at this stage but it is not absolutely necessary (Fig. 3.5).

> **Key point**
> A deficiency of B$_{12}$ or folate will cause distinctive changes in the bone marrow. The difficulty in DNA synthesis leads to premature cell death and ineffective erythropoiesis. Nuclear maturation is delayed, resulting in megaloblastic change.

Table 3.4 Vitamin and antibody levels

	Patient's results	Normal range
Serum B$_{12}$	50 ng/l	150–1000 ng/l (pg/ml)
Red cell folate	200 ng/l of packed red cells	150–1000 ng/l (pg/ml)
Intrinsic factor (IF) antibodies	Positive	
Parietal cell (PC) antibodies	Positive	

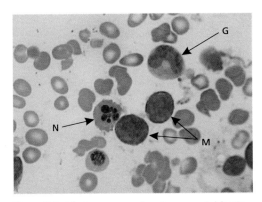

Figure 3.5 A bone marrow showing megaloblastic red cell precursors (M), a 'giant metamyelocyte' (G, a granulocyte precursor) and a red cell precursor with nuclear fragments (N). The maturation of the nucleus is out of synchrony with the cytoplasm.

Q11 Why should she be given folate and B_{12} replacement?

A Giving folate alone to an individual who has B_{12} deficiency may correct the blood findings but result in a worsening of the demyelination, which may be irreversible. Therefore, all patients should receive both B_{12} and folate replacement until the diagnosis becomes clear. A deficiency of B_{12} leads to demyelination of the brain and spinal cord. This does not occur with folate deficiency. The clinical manifestations are confusion and memory loss together with a combination of signs in the lower limbs reflecting demyelination of the posterior and lateral columns of the spinal cord, a syndrome known as sub-acute combined degeneration.

> **Key point**
>
> Early treatment of B_{12} deficiency often results in an improvement in the peripheral neuropathy. The spinal cord abnormalities are not reversible and that is why early diagnosis is so important.

Q12 How do these results help to confirm a suspected diagnosis of B_{12} deficiency?

A The low level of B_{12} with normal red cell folate and positive antibodies confirms B_{12} deficiency and suggests an autoimmune aetiology.

Q13 What is the connection between the low serum potassium level and the B_{12} deficiency?

A The abnormal DNA synthesis affects the cells lining the renal tubules, leading to a potassium-wasting syndrome. This results in low serum potassium.

> **Key point**
>
> When effective treatment with vitamin B_{12} is given there will be a sudden burst of activity in the marrow with many new healthy cells being formed and the serum potassium may fall further leading to sudden death. Therefore, it is important to give early potassium replacement and to monitor potassium levels in the first week of treatment.

Q14 What else in the history is relevant to the diagnosis of an autoimmune disease?

A A family history of other autoimmune disease such as thyroid disease in her sister.

A The reticulocyte count begins to increase within 2–3 days, reflecting the new healthy red cells being released from the marrow. The red cell count will increase within 1–2 weeks and the MCV will return to normal over 4–6 weeks.

A In this age group, pernicious anaemia is the most common cause of B_{12} deficiency; however, other causes include: partial/total gastrectomy, Crohn's disease (with or without ileal resection), blind loop syndromes, tropical sprue and fish tapeworm.

A A test using radioactive isotopes to measure the excretion of B_{12} in the urine is called the Schilling test. It can differentiate between pernicious anaemia and other mechanisms of B_{12} deficiency. The use of radioactive-based tests has become much less frequent with the development of reliable serum assays.

Key point

It is increasingly being recognized that vegans and people in 'old people homes', where dietary protein may be minimal, may develop B_{12} deficiency. It can also be seen occasionally in young people.

A 30-year-old woman was referred from the infertility clinic because she had a raised MCV (macrocytosis). Serum B_{12} was low and IF antibodies were detected. Within 2 months of replacement therapy she became pregnant.

Deficiencies of vitamin B_{12} or folate may be significant contributors to vascular dementia and Alzheimer's disease because of the elevated levels of homocysteine (see diagram of B_{12}/folate interactions, Fig. 3.4).

Can you now construct an algorithm to investigate a patient with pancytopenia?

A Yes.

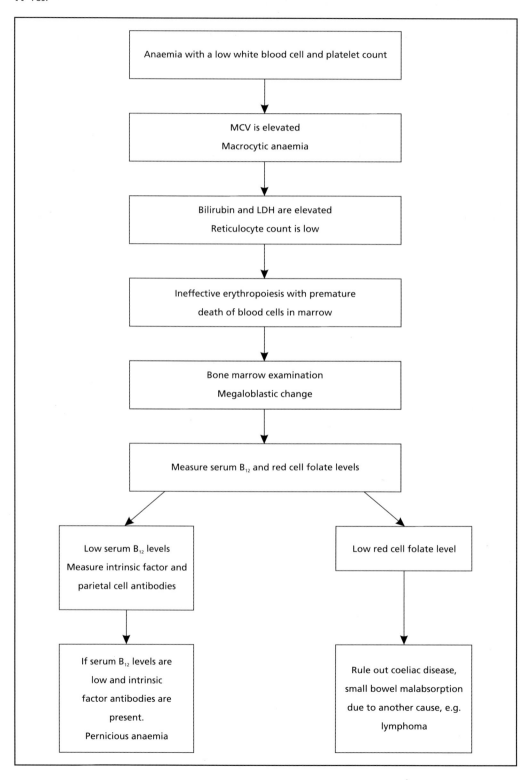

OUTCOME

The patient responded well to vitamin B_{12} replacement with a return of her blood and biochemical tests to normal after 5 weeks. Her mental state improved even more quickly and she enjoyed seeing her grandchildren again.

After 6 months the doctor advised her to take her B_{12} indefinitely as she was very reliable and agreed to come for 6 monthly blood counts and medical checks.

Suggested reading

Chanarin, I. (1990) *The Megaloblastic Anaemias*, 3rd edn. Blackwell Scientific, Oxford.

Wickramasinghe, S.N. (1995) Megaloblastic anaemia. In: *Baillière's Clinical Haematology, International Practice and Research* (ed. S.N. Wickramasinghe), Vol. 8, No. 3, pp. 441–459. Baillière Tindall, Oxford.

Weir, D.G. & Scott, J.M. (1999) Brain function in the elderly: role of vitamin B_{12} and folate. *British Medical Bulletin*, **55**(3), 669–82.

Antony, A.C. (2000) Megaloblastic anemias. In: *Hematology. Basic Principles and Practice* (eds R. Hoffman, E.J. Benz, Jr, S.J. Shattil, B. Furie, H.J. Cohen, L.E. Silberstein & P. McGlave), 3rd edn, pp. 446–85. Churchill Livingstone, New York, USA.

Hoffbrand, A.V., Pettit, J.E. & Moss, P.A.H. (2001) *Essential Haematology*, 4th edn. Blackwell Science, Oxford. See Chapter 4: Megaloblastic anaemias and other macrocytic anaemias.

A young man with weight loss and diarrhoea

A 25-year-old bus driver went to the company doctor in April because he noticed that he was losing weight and had diarrhoea. The patient admitted that he had to tighten his belt by two holes. He did not wear a tie every day but definitely thought that his collar was a little looser.

Q1 How would you evaluate his signs and symptoms?

A Weight loss can be difficult to estimate, as many people do not keep an accurate account of their weight. The fact that he tightened his belt and said that his collar felt loose suggests significant weight loss. The duration of the diarrhoea, its frequency and colour are also important.

Blood and mucus in the stool should be asked about as they could indicate chronic inflammatory bowel disease, diverticular disease or cancer. The latter two, however, are unlikely because of the patient's age. Pale-coloured stools with a foul smell and which are difficult to 'flush away' are suggestive of malabsorption.

He said he had been feeling unwell and noticed the altered bowel habit since Christmas.

Q2 What other condition, which is common in young adults, could present with an altered bowel habit?

A 'Irritable bowel syndrome' typically occurs in young adults. It is often associated with 'stress'.

Q3 What would you do next?

A Take a social and family history.

He was never ill before. He smokes 20 cigarettes per day and only drinks at weekends when he has a 'few pints' on a Friday and Saturday night. He has one brother and one sister, both older than him and they are both very well. His parents are well and he does not know much about his extended family. He lives at home with his parents and eats his main meal with them every day.

Q4 **What should be done next?**

A A physical examination.

On physical examination he was nervous with sweaty palms and a pulse of 100 per minute. Weight loss was apparent because of his loosely fitting clothes. He had pale conjunctivae and palmar creases. His abdomen was soft but no masses or organomegaly were palpable.

Q5 **What should be done next?**

A A full blood count (Table 4.1), blood film (Fig. 4.1) and biochemical screen (Table 4.2).

Table 4.1 Full blood count

	Patient's results	Normal range (male)
Hb	10.0 g/dl	13.5–18.0 g/dl
MCV	105 fl	83–99 fl (μm^3)
MCH	30 pg/cell	26.7–32.5 pg/cell
MCHC	32 g/dl	30.8–34.6 g/dl
RBC	3.0×10^{12}/l	$4.60–5.70 \times 10^{12}$/l (10^6/μl)
WBC	3.5×10^9/l	$4.0–11.0 \times 10^9$/l (10^3/μl)
Platelets	120×10^9/l	$140–450 \times 10^9$/l (10^3/μ)
Reticulocyte count	30×10^9/l	$20–100 \times 10^9$/l (0.2–1.5%)

The blood film (Fig. 4.1) was reported as having oval macrocytes (larger than normal red cells and oval shaped rather than the usual disc), and abnormally shaped cells (poikilocytes). The platelets were decreased in number.

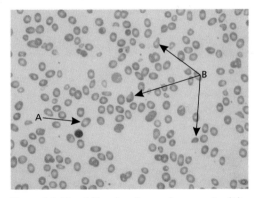

Figure 4.1 Blood film showing oval macrocytes (A) and poikilocytes (B), abnormally shaped red cells.

Q6 **How can you connect the diarrhoea and the blood findings?**

A Macrocytic anaemia with pancytopenia (reduced white cells and platelets), diarrhoea and weight loss suggest a malabsorption syndrome.

A The reticulocyte count. A high reticulocyte count means the marrow is responding by making more red cells and a low reticulocyte count means that the marrow is incapable of responding.

> **Key point**
>
> In this case the low reticulocyte count and the low red blood cell count. (Table 4.1) suggest a production problem in the marrow. The biochemical screen also revealed some abnormalities (Table 4.2).

Table 4.2 Biochemical results

	Patient's results	Normal range
Bilirubin	22 µmol/l	0–17 µmol/l (0.3–1.1 mg/dl)
Lactic dehydrogenase (LDH)	3000 IU/l	230–450 IU/l

Q8 How can the biochemical findings be explained?

A The bilirubin and LDH may come from prematurely destroyed red cells. Bilirubin is present in the unconjugated state before passing through the liver, where it is conjugated. Thus, the unconjugated bilirubin will be elevated in haemolysis. However, in clinical practice, the total bilirubin is commonly measured. Thus, the biochemical profile enhances the suspicion of a 'production' problem in the marrow.

Q9 What mechanisms might cause the marrow to produce red cells that are too large?

A Deficiencies of the vitamins B_{12} or folate affect DNA synthesis in all dividing cells and since the bone marrow contains rapidly dividing cells, marrow production will be an early casualty. Abnormalities in the bone marrow are reflected in the white and red cell counts, which are readily available.

Q10 What should be done next?

A Serum B_{12} and red cell folate levels (Table 4.3). Deficiencies of either of these vitamins can cause macrocytosis and pancytopenia.

Table 4.3 Serum B_{12} and red cell folate

	Patient's results	Normal range
Red cell folate	75 ng/l of packed red cells	150–1000 µg/l (pg/ml)
Serum B_{12}	180 ng/l	150–1000 ng/l (pg/ml)
Serum ferritin	5.0 µg/l	20–300 µg/l (pg/ml)

A A low folate would suggest a malabsorption syndrome or a dietary deficiency. He lives at home and eats with his parents so a dietary deficiency is unlikely.

Q12 If a dietary deficiency is unlikely, what diseases cause folate malabsorption?

A Coeliac disease, secondary to Gliadin toxicity, a component of wheat, interferes with the absorption of folate by causing severe damage to the lining of the small bowel. Rapid turnover of the cells lining the small bowel in coeliac disease, which are shed into the bowel lumen, also contributes to the low folate levels.

A childhood history of diarrhoea or a family history of malabsorption should increase your suspicion of coeliac disease. Ask him to find out if he had been investigated as a child for diarrhoea or 'failure to thrive' or if any of his family had been diagnosed with coeliac disease?

Q13 What should be done next?

A Refer the patient for specialist investigation because of the macrocytosis and pancytopenia.

The haematologist agreed that the presence of macrocytosis and pancytopenia warranted further investigation. He carried out a bone marrow aspirate, which revealed megaloblastic change (Figs 4.2–4.4). Figure 4.2 shows a bone marrow aspirate showing 'megaloblastic' red cell precursors and 'giant' white cell precursors. The red cell precursors exhibit fragmented nuclei and

delayed nuclear maturation. Figure 4.3 shows a bone marrow stained for iron, which is absent. In coeliac disease there is a combination of iron and folate deficiency. Figure 4.4 shows a megaloblastic bone marrow (vitamin B_{12} deficiency). Iron is usually increased because of the ineffective erythropoiesis and increased rate of apoptosis. Iron is seen as a green stain.

In view of the diarrhoea and weight loss he also ordered a jejunal biopsy (Figs 4.5 and 4.6), which showed features of coeliac disease. Figure 4.5 is an endoscopic jejunal biopsy showing blunted villi and an inflammatory infiltrate of lymphocytes.

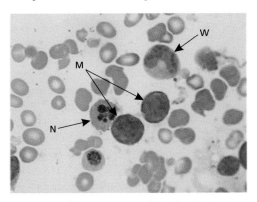

Figure 4.2 A bone marrow aspirate showing 'megaloblastic' red cell precursors (M) and 'giant' white cell precursors (W). The red cell precursors exhibit fragmented nuclei and delayed nuclear maturation (N).

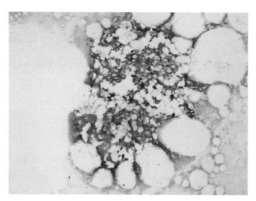

Figure 4.3 A bone marrow stained for iron, which is absent. In coeliac disease, there is a combination of iron and folate deficiency.

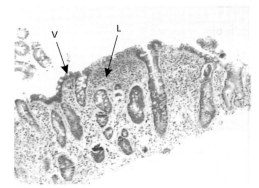

Figure 4.5 An endoscopic jejunal biopsy showing blunted villi (V) and an inflammatory infiltrate of lymphocytes (L).

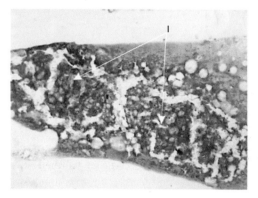

Figure 4.4 A megaloblastic bone marrow (folate deficiency). Iron is usually increased because of the ineffective erythropoiesis and increased rate of apoptosis. Iron is seen as a green stain, I.

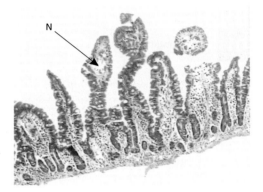

Figure 4.6 An endoscopic jejunal biopsy showing normal villi (N) and no lymphocytic infiltrate.

Q14 How can the megaloblastic changes in the marrow be explained?

A A deficiency of folate leads to ineffective DNA synthesis.

> **Key point**
>
> Deficiency of folate causes marrow damage because 5,10-methylene THF is a coenzyme in the synthesis of thymidylate (which is required for pyrimidine and DNA synthesis) and of S-adenosylmethionine (which controls DNA production by its methylation) (see Fig. 4.7).

Folates are compounds derived from pteroylglutamic acid. The daily requirements are about 100 µg and a 'normal' diet supplies about 150 µg/day. Folates are present in most green vegetables and liver but are partially destroyed by cooking. Folates are absorbed through the upper small bowel and body stores last for only 3–4 months. This is in complete contrast to B_{12}, where the body stores last for years. All dietary folates are converted to methyltetrahydrofolate (THF) by the small bowel. Folates are involved in many important biochemical reactions needing single carbon transfer.

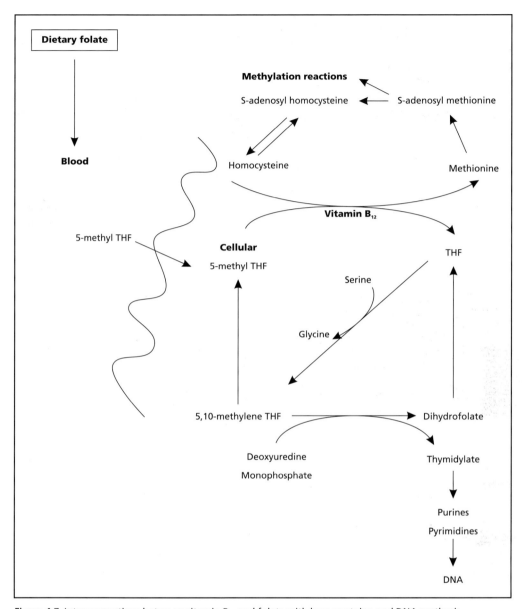

Figure 4.7 Interconnections between vitamin B$_{12}$ and folate with homocysteine and DNA synthesis.

The tissue transglutaminase (tTG) antibody was elevated at 20 μ/ml (normal <5 μ/ml), which together with the appearances of the jejunal biopsy, confirmed a diagnosis of coeliac disease.

Q15 What other diseases might be confused with coeliac disease?

A Tropical sprue, enteric (bowel) infections or lymphomas can present similarly.

Q16 Can you now construct an algorithm to help in the diagnosis of a patient with folate deficiency?

A Yes.

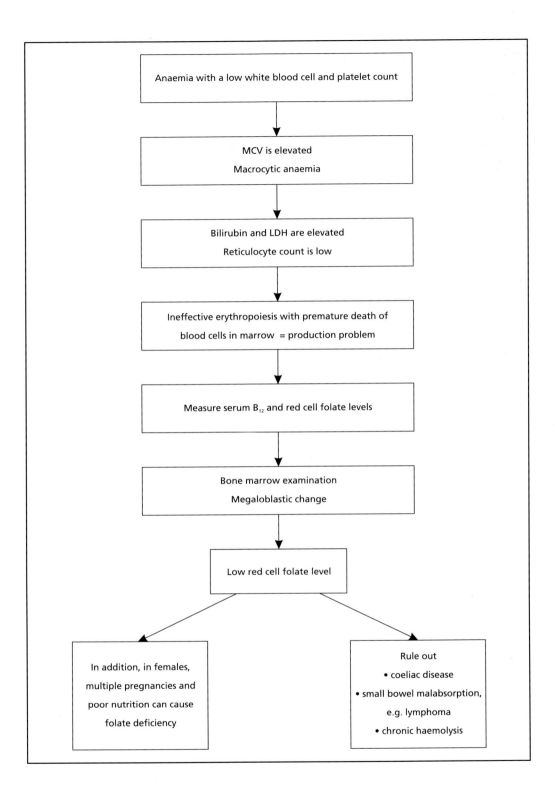

A A deficiency of folate in the mother at the time of conception increases the risk of neural tube defects in the foetus (spina bifida).

Key point

Individuals who have the common mutation in 5,10-methylene tetrahydrofolate (THF) reductase (677C-T) have a greater risk of deficiency and of giving birth to children with neural tube defects. Dietary supplementation with folic acid reduces the incidence of neural tube defects and is now recommended for all females contemplating pregnancy.

OUTCOME

A diagnosis of coeliac disease was made and the patient was placed on a gluten-free diet. He was given iron and folate supplements for 3 months. He was advised to stay on the diet for the rest of his life to minimize the risk of developing a lymphoma in his small bowel. His blood counts recovered, his bowel habit returned to normal and he returned to work 6 weeks later.

Key point

Failure to adhere to the diet causes continual damage to the bowel and can result in the development of a lymphoma.

Suggested reading

Kelly, C.P., Feighery, C.F., Gallagher, R.B. & Weir, D.G. (1990) Diagnosis and treatment of gluten-sensitive enteropathy. *Advances in Internal Medicine*, **35**, 341–63.

Antony, A.C. (2000) Megaloblastic anemias. In: *Hematology. Basic Principles and Practice* (eds R. Hoffman, E.J. Benz, Jr, S.J. Shattil, B. Furie, H.J. Cohen, L.E. Silberstein & P. McGlave), 3rd edn, pp. 446–85. Churchill Livingstone, New York, USA.

Hoffbrand, A.V., Pettit, J.E. & Moss, P.A.H. (2001) *Essential Haematology*, 4th edn. Blackwell Science, Oxford. See Chapter 4: Megaloblastic anaemias and other macrocytic anaemias.

Molloy, A.M. & Scott, J.M. (2001) Folates and prevention of disease. *Public Health and Nutrition*, **4** (2B), 601–9.

Farrell, R.J. & Kelly, C. (2002) Coeliac sprue. *New England Journal of Medicine*, **364** (3), 180–8.

A young man with abdominal pain and jaundice

A 30-year-old male schoolteacher telephoned the surgery for an appointment. He said that he had been feeling very tired for the last 2 weeks and that his wife remarked to him that she thought he had yellow eyes. He also said that he had pain in his stomach, on and off, for a week.

Q1 What might be going on?

A His yellow eyes suggest that he is jaundiced and his fatigue is obviously significant as it was the first thing he mentioned. He might have hepatitis or gallstones, or it could be a reaction to a medication. It is appropriate to give him an early appointment.

Q2 What general observations should be made?

A Does he look ill or in distress with his pain? Has he has lost weight? Is he jaundiced?

He looks well and is not distressed. He is not in pain and does not appear to have lost weight. His sclerae are mildly icteric (jaundiced).

Q3 What questions should be asked initially?

A Has the fatigue been getting worse? Is the abdominal pain becoming more severe, lasting longer or associated with any other symptoms such as nausea, vomiting or loss of appetite?

On closer questioning it was clear that fatigue had been a feature of this man's life. While at school he had not participated in contact sports because he always felt 'a little under the weather.' There had been at least two episodes of 'hepatitis' when he was 7 and 9 years old.

Q4 Was this 'infective hepatitis' or could his past episodes of jaundice be related to his present complaints?

A He could have had 'infective hepatitis' but the fact that it occurred twice should make you suspect another explanation.

Hepatitis is an infection of the liver. It is commonly caused by a virus and usually is a mild self-limiting illness. The most likely cause of infective hepatitis in a child would be hepatitis A. Other viruses that cause hepatitis include hepatitis B and C but these types of infection would be much less likely in an otherwise healthy child.

A A detailed medical, travel and drug history. Ask about any episodes of jaundice in family members.

His holidays had been in Europe and Australia. There were no other problems except an appendicectomy when he was 5 years. He had one younger brother who was well. His mother was alive and well and his father had died 2 years ago of a 'heart attack'. He had no children. There was no family history of jaundice. He was not taking medication and denied use of illegal substances.

Eye examination confirmed the presence of jaundice and his spleen was palpable 2 cm below his left costal margin. There was some tenderness in the right upper quadrant but his abdomen was soft.

A He could have some form of congenital haemolytic anaemia (premature destruction of his red cells) with gallstones. This would account for the recurrent episodes of jaundice, enlarged spleen and abdominal pain.

Other causes of a large spleen, in a patient of this age, include Hodgkin's disease, non-Hodgkin's lymphoma, portal hypertension, chronic my-eloid leukaemia and acquired forms of haemolytic anaemia. None of these diseases would be likely to cause the combination of symptoms and signs which this patient exhibits.

> **Key point**
> Importantly, the patient looks and feels well, making an underlying malignancy unlikely.

A A full blood count, blood film, biochemical screen, urinalysis and blood pressure. A chest radiograph and an ultrasound examination of his abdomen should be ordered.

His blood pressure was 125/80 mmHg. His urine contained urobilinogen.

He should be advised to stay off work until the investigations are completed (Table 5.1 and Fig. 5.1).

Table 5.1 Full blood count

	Patient's results	Normal range
Hb	12.5 g/dl	13.5–18.0 g/dl
MCV	103 fl	83–99 fl (μm^3)
MCH	30 pg/cell	27–32 pg/cell
MCHC	36 g/dl	30–36 g/dl
RBC	6.0×10^{12}/l	4.5–6.5×10^{12}/l (10^6/μl)
WBC	10.5×10^9/l	4.0–11.0×10^9/l (10^3/μl)

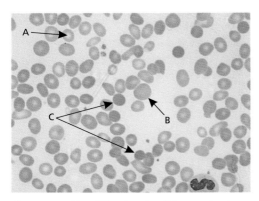

Figure 5.1 A blood film showing (A) normal red cells with central pallor, (B) polychromasia (grey/blue cells synthesising Hb) and (C) spherocytes which are smaller and denser than normal red cells and have no central pallor.

Q8 How can the blood results be interpreted?

A He is anaemic and has a high MCV (macrocytosis) and spherocytes. He could have haemolytic anaemia.

Other conditions which could cause anaemia and macrocytosis include vitamin B_{12} or folate deficiency or liver disease.

Q9 What test could help to confirm your suspicion of haemolysis?

A A reticulocyte count, bilirubin and lactic dehydrogenase (Table 5.2).

Table 5.2 Reticulocyte count and biochemical abnormalities

	Patient's results	Normal range
Reticulocyte	130×10^9/l	$50–100 \times 10^9$/l (0.5–1.5%)
Bilirubin	25 µmol/l	0–17 µmol/l (0.3–1.1 mg/dl)
Lactic dehydrogenase (LDH)	650 IU/l	230–450 IU/l

Q10 How do these findings help to make a diagnosis?

A The elevated reticulocyte count suggests that the bone marrow is producing young red cells in response to the anaemia. These young red cells, reticulocytes, are larger than mature red cells, which explain the raised MCV. The elevated bilirubin and LDH and the urobilinogen in the urine are the result of red cell destruction (Fig. 5.2). The level of indirect (unconjugated) bilirubin is elevated in haemolysis. The spherocytes indicate a congenital or acquired membrane defect.

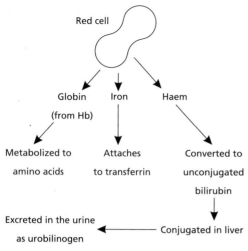

Red cell

Globin   Iron   Haem

(from Hb)

Metabolized to   Attaches   Converted to

amino acids   to transferrin   unconjugated

bilirubin

Excreted in the urine   ←   Conjugated in liver

as urobilinogen

Figure 5.2 A diagrammatic representation of the breakdown of Hb after the red cell dies. Normally, red cells are broken down in the reticuloendothelial system (liver, spleen, and bone marrow) after 120 days in the circulation. The haem, which is converted to bilirubin, can cause jaundice and pigment gallstones.

> **Key point**
> In this case it is likely that the patient never had 'infective hepatitis' but instead had an episode of jaundice associated with haemolysis.

Q11   What should the patient and his wife be told?

A He probably has a congenital disorder of his red cells, leading to their premature destruction. He should be referred to the next available outpatient haematology clinic but this was not an emergency. The discomfort in his right upper quadrant is probably due to gallstones and he might need to have his gall-bladder removed.

Q12   What medication should he be offered and why?

A Folic acid should be prescribed.

> **Key point**
> Chronic haemolysis increases the requirement for folate, which is a major coenzyme in nucleic acid synthesis. Depletion of folate will inhibit the production of new red cells and the anaemia will become more marked.

Q13 What might suggest that the patient was becoming depleted in folic acid?

A The reticulocyte count would be reduced and the anaemia would become more severe.

The patient was seen by a haematologist the following week. She confirmed the history and physical findings. The chest radiography was normal and the ultrasound of the abdomen (Fig. 5.3) confirmed an enlarged spleen.

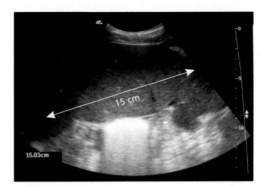

Figure 5.3 Ultrasound examination of the left upper quadrant of the abdomen. The dark grey area (under the arrow) represents the spleen, which is enlarged measuring 15 cm (normal 11–12 cm). This test uses sound waves to 'image' the internal organs without the use of radiation.

Q14 What further tests should she order?

A A direct antiglobulin test (Coomb's test).

This test detects the presence of autoantibody on the red blood cell surface (see case 6 for a full explanation of the antiglobulin test).

The direct antiglobulin test was negative, indicating that the patient did not have an acquired autoimmune haemolytic anaemia (AIHA).

Q15 What further test could explain the mechanism of haemolysis?

A An osmotic fragility test (Figs 5.4 and 5.5), which measures the ability of red cells to resist osmotic shock.

The result indicated that the patient's red cells were less resistant to osmotic shock than normal red cells, which was consistent with a diagnosis of a congenital disorder of the red cell 'cytoskeleton', hereditary spherocytosis syndrome.

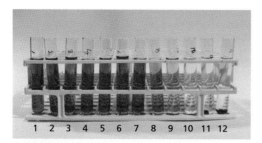

Figure 5.4 The osmotic fragility test, which measures the ability of red cells to resist osmotic shock (resistance to rupture when incubated in saline solutions). As normal red cells are biconcave discs they can resist rupture better than spherocytes because they have a larger surface area to volume ratio. This is reflected by the amount of Hb released when red cells are incubated in different solutions of saline and comparing normal with the patient's sample. Tube 12 contains normal saline and no haemolysis is expected. As the numbers go down to 1 the saline becomes hypotonic and there is a gradual increase in cell rupture and release of Hb.

Key point

A biconcave disc (normal red cell) will change its shape to a sphere when there is a reduction in the ratio of surface area to volume. There are two basic mechanisms to account for this shape change. Congenital disorders which lead to structural changes in the red blood cell 'cytoskeleton' will result in an abnormal spherical shape, the so-called 'hereditary spherocytosis syndrome'. Acquired autoimmune diseases, where antibodies become attached to the red blood cell membrane and are subsequently phagocytosed in the spleen, result in a loss of surface area and formation of a sphere (autoimmune haemolytic anaemia, AIHA) (case 6).

Thus, two entirely different mechanisms can result in formation of spherocytes and premature red blood cell destruction.

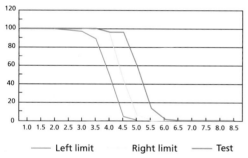

— Left limit   Right limit   — Test

Figure 5.5 The green line is a measure of the degree of the patient's red cell rupture at the various concentrations of saline corresponding to tubes 1 to 12 (normal levels are between the blue and yellow lines).

Q16   What other investigation might help to confirm the diagnosis?

A Flow cytometric analysis will confirm the abnormal cytoskeletal membrane structure.

Key point

The history of recurrent jaundice together with the evidence of haemolysis and a negative direct antiglobulin (Coomb's) test is indicative of the hereditary spherocytosis syndrome.

A Patients with chronic haemolysis may develop multiple small gallstones (Fig. 5.6), which may cause abdominal pain or obstruct the common bile duct.

These gallstones are the result of increased red cell destruction and increased haem metabolism to bilirubin. They are called pigment stones. If a small gallstone becomes impacted in the common bile duct, obstructive jaundice will occur and the elevation in bilirubin will be primarily direct (conjugated).

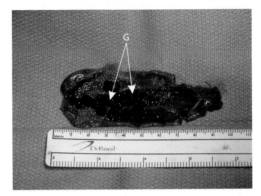

Figure 5.6 Gall-bladder, removed at surgery, with multiple pigment stones.

A Yes.

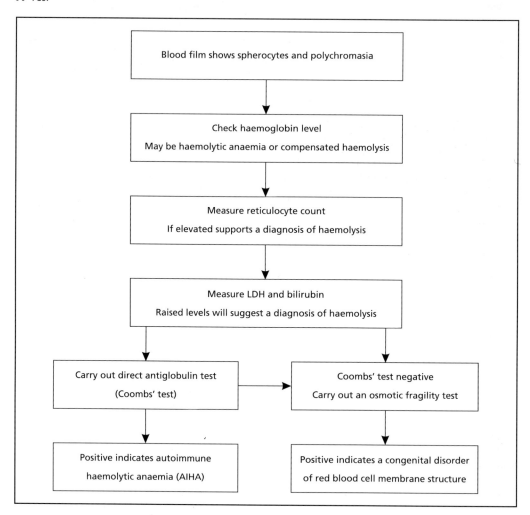

OUTCOME

Initially, he was treated conservatively and given folic acid daily. His jaundice cleared but recurred 3 and 6 months later. He also had three episodes of right upper abdominal pain. Following vaccination against pneumococcus and *Haemophilus influenzae* his gall-bladder, because of symptomatic stones (Fig. 5.6) and spleen (because of recurrent anaemia) (Fig. 5.7) were removed and he was given life-long prophylaxis with penicillin.

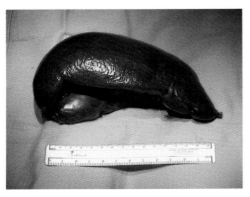

Figure 5.7 Enlarged spleen, removed at surgery.

> **Key point**
> His reticulocyte count returned to normal within 3 days of surgery. Removal of the spleen will _not_ correct the underlying red cell membrane defect but will allow the red cell lifespan to return, almost to normal. Splenectomy is NOT carried out on young children and should only be undertaken for recurrent anaemia and symptoms.

Suggested reading

Hassoun, H. & Palek, J. (1996) Hereditary spherocytosis: a review of the clinical and molecular aspects of the disease. *Blood Reviews*, **10** (3), 129–47.

Antony, A.C. (2000) Red cell membrane disorders. In: *Hematology. Basic Principles and Practice* (eds R. Hoffman, E.J. Benz, Jr, S.J. Shattil, B. Furie, H.J. Cohen, L.E. Silberstein & P. McGlave), 3rd edn, pp. 546–610. Churchill Livingstone, New York, USA.

Hoffbrand, A.V., Pettit, J.E. & Moss, P.A.H. (2001) *Essential Haematology*, 4th edn. Blackwell Science, Oxford. See Chapter 5: Haemolytic anaemias.

Gallagher, P.G. & Jarolim, P. (2000) In: *Hematology: Basic Principles and Practice* (eds R. Hoffman, E.J. Benz, Jr, S.J. Shattil, B. Furie, H.J. Cohen, L.E. Silberstein & P. McGlave), 3rd edn, pp. 546–610. Churchill Livingstone, New York, USA.

Roper, D. Layton, M. & Lewis, S.M. (2001) *Dacie & Lewis Practical Haematology* (eds S.M. Lewis, B.J. Bain and I. Bates), 9th edn, pp. 167–98. Churchill Livingstone, New York, USA.

Delaunay, J. (2003) Red cell membrane and erythropoiesis genetic defects. *The Hematology Journal*, **4**, 225–32.

An elderly man unable to take his dog for a walk

A 70-year-old Caucasian man went to his family doctor. He had had a Jack Russell terrier for 10 years and usually walked him for 30–40 minutes in the evening. For the last few weeks he has noticed he was short of breath after about 10 minutes. This symptom had been getting worse – to the point that he no longer feels he wants to walk his dog.

Q1 What might explain his symptoms?

A A change in work or recreation patterns is always suggestive of disease.

Q2 What question(s) might define when the symptoms began?

A Were you well before ...? (Use a well-known public holiday, e.g. Christmas, or a national event.)

Q3 What associated symptoms should be enquired about?

A Symptoms relating to the respiratory or cardiovascular systems. A history of previous episodes of shortness of breath, a cough productive of sputum or blood (haemoptysis), wheeze or chest tightness or discomfort on exertion. Symptoms such as ankle swelling or waking suddenly from sleep with shortness of breath suggest a cardiac cause.

Ask him if he has ever been treated for high blood pressure, angina, asthma or chronic bronchitis. Review his medications and his smoking habits.

The patient states that he has been well all his life and 'never goes near a doctor'. He denies a history of the symptoms about which he has been questioned. He is a non-smoker.

A Take a full history, including a family and personal history of tuberculosis. A positive family history or contact with a person with tuberculosis could put him at risk. Travel to areas where unusual infections are present should be noted.

His holidays had always been taken in Europe. He had no known contact with anyone with tuberculosis.

Q5 **What should be done next?**

A A full physical examination.

His blood pressure was 125/80 mmHg and his respiratory rate was 20/min. His sclerae were jaundiced (icteric) and he was pale. His pulse was regular but slightly fast at 100 beats/min.

His heart size was normal and no murmurs were present, but he had fine crackles at both his lung bases on inspiration. He had no lymphadenopathy but his spleen was palpable 3 cm below his left costal margin. He had bilateral pitting ankle oedema.

Q6 **What do these signs suggest?**

A His pallor and jaundice suggest anaemia and liver disease, haemolysis or ineffective erythropoiesis (cells dying prematurely in the marrow). His rapid pulse, inspiratory crackles and ankle swelling suggest mild heart failure and his large spleen, an unexpected finding, suggests a haematological or infectious component to his symptoms.

Q7 **What investigations should be carried out?**

A A full blood count and reticulocyte count (Table 6.1), blood film (Fig. 6.1) and biochemical screen should be done.

Table 6.1 Full blood count

	Patient's results	Normal range (male)
Hb	5.8 g/dl	13.5–18.0 g/dl
MCV	121 fl	83.0–99.0 fl (μm^3)
WBC	7.9×10^9/l	$4.0–11.0 \times 10^9$/l (10^3/μl)
Platelets	450×10^9/l	$140–450 \times 10^9$/l (10^3/μl)
Red cell count	1.58×10^{12}/l	$4.60–5.70 \times 10^{12}$/l (10^6/ml)
Reticulocytes	320×10^9/l	$20–100 \times 10^9$/l (0.2–1.5%)

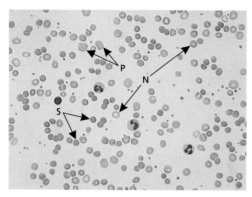

Figure 6.1 A blood film showing normal red cells (N), spherocytes (S) and polychromasia (P).

Red cells are biconcave discs and when looked at on a blood film appear to have an area of central pallor. Most of the haemoglobin is around the edge of the cell and not in the middle, hence the appearance. Spherocytes are almost completely spherical but in a two-dimensional view will appear as small dense cells without central pallor. The haemoglobin is equally distributed throughout the cell. The polychromasia or blue/grey colour of the red cells reflects the presence of ribosomes and haemoglobin synthesis. These young red cells are called reticulocytes. They are present in the peripheral blood in small numbers (50–100 × 10^9/l). If there is premature removal of red cells from the circulation (due to haemolysis or bleeding) this will be reflected by an increase in the number of reticulocytes found in the peripheral blood as a compensatory measure.

Q8   How can the results of the blood count be interpreted?

A The low Hb means the patient is anaemic and the low red cell count suggests there are production problems in the marrow or that red cells have a shortened lifespan in the peripheral blood. The elevated MCV reflects the presence of an increased number of reticulocytes, which are large. This would indicate bleeding or haemolysis.

Q9   What is the significance of spherocytes in the blood?

A Spherocytes indicate a congenital or acquired alteration in the surface area to volume ratio of the red cells.

Loss of red cell membrane alters the ratio of cell surface area to volume and this results in the shape change. Red cells are normally very plastic and the biconcave shape facilitates reversible shape change as the cells traverse small blood vessels and the cords of the spleen. Spherocytes are inherently less plastic and have much more difficulty traversing apertures <8.0 μm in diameter.

Q10 By what mechanisms can normal red cell biconcave discs change into spherocytes?

A Inherited abnormalities of red cell membrane, which interfere with the structure/function of the spectrin/actin complex (cytoskeleton), give rise to spherocytes, the so-called hereditary spherocytosis syndrome. Attachment of autoantibodies, with or without complement, to the red cell membrane results in phagocytosis of the attached antibody/complement by macrophages with subsequent loss of red cell membrane (Fig. 6.2).

> **Key point**
> The mechanism of spherocyte formation cannot be ascertained from the blood film appearances.

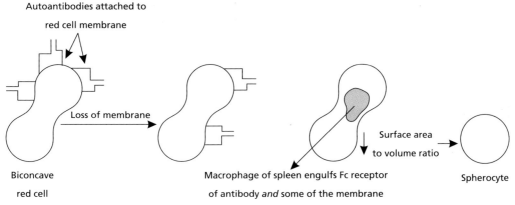

Figure 6.2 A diagram showing autoantibodies attached to the red cell membrane. Thus, autoantibodies and endothelial cells in the spleen engulf some of the red cell membrane. Membrane is lost and a spherocyte is formed.

Q11 What tests can differentiate the mechanism of spherocyte formation?

A The direct antiglobulin test, also known as the Coombs' test (DCT).

Q12 How does the DCT differentiate between the mechanisms?

A The DCT detects the presence of autoantibodies (usually IgG) or complement (usually C3d) on the red cell membrane.

A reagent called the Coombs' reagent is used. This reagent is made by immunizing rabbits with human serum. The rabbit responds by making antibodies.

Q13 What components of serum does the rabbit make antibodies against?

A IgG and complement.

Q21 Why should blood transfusion be avoided?

A The antigens on the transfused red cells may stimulate further production of antibody in the recipient's plasma and increase the rate of haemolysis.

Key point

Give folic acid orally. Patients who have haemolysis may become deficient in folic acid because of the excessive demand by the bone marrow to make new red cells leading to a worsening of the anaemia. A falling reticulocyte count with a further fall in the Hb is suggestive of folate deficiency.

Q22 Which other types of autoantibodies can cause haemolysis?

A Antibodies of the IgM class, so-called cold antibodies, can bind to the red cell surface and always bind complement.

The patient may experience acrocyanosis (purple discoloration of the extremities) in cold weather due to clumping of red cells in the circulation.

Treatment point

Recently, patients with chronic haemolytic anaemia which fails to respond to corticosteroids have been successfully treated with anti-CD20 antibody.

A Yes.

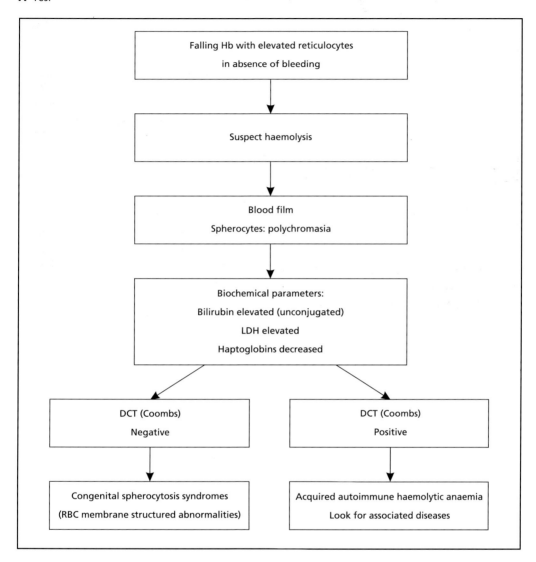

OUTCOME

The patient was given oral corticosteroids and folic acid supplements. Anti-fungal prophylaxis and proton pump inhibitors were prescribed to counteract the major toxicities of corticosteroids and his blood glucose was monitored carefully. No underlying disease was detected and his Hb returned to normal in 4 weeks.

Suggested reading

Dacie, Sir J. (1995) In: *The Haemolytic Anaemias*, Vol. 4. *Secondary or Symptomatic Haemolytic Anaemias* (ed. Sir John Dacie), 3rd edn. Churchill Livingstone, Edinburgh, UK.

Schwartz, R.S., Beakman, E.H. & Silberstein, L.E. (2000) Autoimmune haemolytic anemias. In: *Hematology. Basic Principles and Practice* (eds R. Hoffman, E.J. Benz, Jr, S.J. Shattil, B. Furie, H.J. Cohen, L.E. Silberstein & P. McGlave), 3rd edn, pp. 611–30. Churchill Livingstone, New York, USA.

Hoffbrand, A.V., Pettit, J.E. & Moss, P.A.H. (2001) *Essential Haematology*, 4th edn. Blackwell Science, Oxford. See Chapter 5: Haemolytic anaemias.

Gupta, N., Kavuru, S., Patel, D., Janson, D., Driscoll, N., Ahmed, S. & Rai, K.R. (2002) Rituximab-based chemotherapy for steroid-refractory autoimmune haemolytic anemia of chronic lymphocytic leukaemia. *Leukemia*, **16** (10), 2092–5.

A young Nigerian man with shortness of breath and anaemia

Ola, a 35-year-old computer analyst from Nigeria, presented to the Accident and Emergency Department complaining of chest pain and shortness of breath for 48 hours. He was ill and distressed. His pulse rate was 120/min (75–90) and his blood pressure was 140/90 mmHg (120/80). He was tachypnoeic (breathing quickly) at a rate of 35/min (12–16). His oxygen saturation was 82% (normal >96%). He was jaundiced and his temperature was 38°C. He was given oxygen, pain relief with morphine and hydrated intravenously.

When he was more comfortable he said that he had been diagnosed as having sickle cell anaemia when he was a child. He could not remember much about his childhood illness but he had many admissions to hospital for 'painful crises' and had become dependent on opioid analgesics (narcotic pain-relieving drugs).

Q1 What investigations should be done immediately?

A A full blood count (Table 7.1), a blood film (Fig. 7.1), a biochemical screen (Table 7.2) and a chest radiograph (Fig. 7.2).

The blood film (Fig. 7.1) showed 'sickle' shaped red cells.

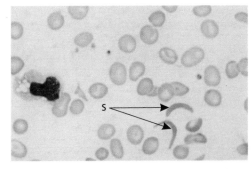

Figure 7.1 A blood film, showing 'sickle cells' (S).

Table 7.1 Full blood count

	Patient's results	Normal range (male)
Hb	6.70 g/dl	13.5–18.0 g/dl
WBC	18.7 × 10⁹/l	4.0–11.0 × 10^9/l (10^3/μl)
Platelets	343 × 10⁹/l	140–450 × 10^9/l (10^3/μl)
MCV	85.0 fl	83.0–99.0 fl (μm³)
MCHC	36.0 g/dl	30.8–34.6 g/dl
Red cell count	2.72 × 10¹²/l	4.60–5.70 × 10^{12}/l (10^6/μl)
Neutrophils	14.8 × 10⁹/l	2.0–7.5 × 10^9/l (10^3/μl)
Lymphocytes	2.0 × 10⁹/l	1.5–3.5 × 10^9/l (10^3/μl)

A The patient is severely anaemic. The presence of abnormally 'sickle' shaped cells in the blood suggests 'sickle cell' anaemia. The raised MCHC is due to the 'dehydration' of the red cells. The raised white cell count is probably due to infection.

Adults normally have haemoglobin A in their red cells. This haemoglobin is made up of two α and two β globin chains together with the 'haem' or iron-containing moiety.

> **Key point**
> Haemoglobin is normally in solution within the red blood cell.

A large number of congenital diseases exist in which an abnormal gene encodes for an abnormal Hb. If the amino acid 'substitution' results in an alteration in the function of the haemoglobin molecule then disease may occur. The most well-known disease is 'sickle cell disease' in which the substitution of a single amino acid, valine for glutamic acid, in the β chain results in reduced solubility of the haemoglobin molecule. When oxygen concentrations are reduced the haemoglobin 'polymerizes', i.e. comes out of solution, and causes the red cell to become 'stiff' and change its shape into a 'sickle' cell. This leads to obstruction (vaso-occlusion) of blood vessels and infarction (death) of the distal tissue. It also results in premature destruction of red cells (haemolysis), causing anaemia.

A The reticulocyte count and the biochemical screen (Table 7.2).

Table 7.2 Reticulocyte count and biochemical results

	Patient's results	Normal range
Reticulocyte count	275 × 10⁹/l	50–100 × 10⁹/l (0.5–1.5%)
Bilirubin	39 μmol/l	0–17 μmol/l (0.3–1.1 mg/dl)
Lactic dehydrogenase (LDH)	524 IU/l	230–450 IU/l

A The raised reticulocyte count reflects the release of young red blood cells into the circulation and the raised LDH reflects red cell destruction.

Both of these findings support a diagnosis of haemolysis.

A The most likely diagnosis is sickle cell disease and a 'chest syndrome' based upon new pulmonary infiltrates with fever, cough and chest pain. It may be precipitated by an infection. The history, anaemia and abnormally shaped cells in the blood, together with the evidence of haemolysis and the chest signs and symptoms, all support the diagnosis.

Q6 What should be done next?

A The patient should be admitted to a haematology ward.

He remained hypoxaemic with an oxygenation of 88% (normal >96%) and his chest radiograph was abnormal (Fig. 7.2).

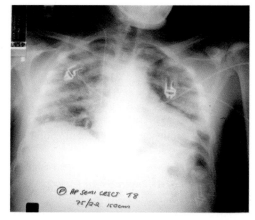

Figure 7.2 Chest radiograph showing bilateral pulmonary infiltrates.

Q7 What other treatment should be considered?

A A blood transfusion might help because he is anaemic and his oxygen-carrying capacity is compromised.

Q8 What are the potential problems associated with red cell transfusion in patients with sickle cell disease?

A There are a number of potential problems.

He has had numerous previous hospitalizations and blood transfusions. Therefore, he may have developed alloantibodies. This will delay the transfusion, as compatible blood must be found.

The distribution of blood group antigens on the red cells of Nigerians is different to that found in Europeans, therefore it may be difficult to find compatible red cells (red cells with the same antigens as the patient's).

In some cases frozen red cells will be required from a blood bank from donors with similar red cell antigens to the patient.

Iron overload may be a problem unless treated with chelating agents.

Q9 What is the aim of the blood transfusion?

A To increase the haemoglobin to approximately 10.0 g/dl, and therefore to decrease the level of abnormal haemoglobin (Hb S) in the circulation.

Q10 What will influence the spectrum of clinical problems experienced by individuals with sickle cell disease?

A The clinical signs and symptoms depend on the ethnic origin of the individual (sickle cell disease is less severe in people from the Middle East than in West Africans).

The signs and symptoms will also vary because many patients have a second mutation in the haemoglobin molecule, which can protect against the tendency of the haemoglobin to 'sickle'.

The level of haemoglobin F (foetal haemoglobin) in the red blood cells in some patients is raised and this protects against 'sickling'. This may be because of a 'genetic adaptation'.

> **Key point**
> Infection with malaria is common in areas where sickle cell disease is prevalent and elevated levels of haemoglobin F can protect red cells from damage caused by malaria parasites.

Q11 What else can influence the degree of 'sickling'?

A The degree of 'sickling' will depend on whether the patient has inherited one or two abnormal (haemoglobin S) alleles.

If one normal and one haemoglobin S allele have been inherited the individual will be a heterozygote and have NO signs and symptoms of sickle cell disease (sickle cell trait). If two abnormal haemoglobin S alleles are inherited the individual is a homozygote and will have all the problems associated with sickle cell disease.

> **Key point**
> Under conditions of severe hypoxia some individuals with sickle trait may develop signs of 'sickling' in their red cells.

Q12 What tests should be done to clarify the diagnosis and why these tests in particular?

A A screening test called the 'Sickledex' (Fig. 7.3) will identify haemoglobin S. Electrophoresis of the haemoglobin will separate haemoglobin S from normal adult haemoglobin (Fig. 7.4). This test will distinguish sickle cell trait (a heterozygote) from sickle cell disease (a homozygote). Different haemoglobins can be separated depending on their charge and the pH of the gel. Note: in an alkaline pH Hb S and Hb D are not separated (Table 7.3), whereas in an acid pH Hb A and Hb S are easily identified.

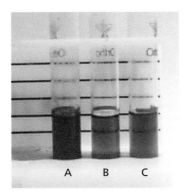

Figure 7.3 turbidity caused by Hb S when a reducing agent is added to the blood.

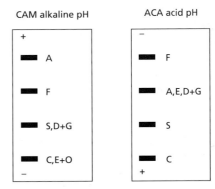

Figure 7.4 The separation of different haemoglobins by electrophoresis.

Q13 What other abnormal haemoglobins occur?

A There are a number of mutant haemoglobins (Table 7.3) that reflect various amino acid substitutions in the Hb molecule.

Table 7.3 Common haemoglobin variants

	Homozygote	Heterozygote	Country of origin
Haemoglobin E*	EE Mild anaemia MCV reduced Target cells	AE Normal Hb level MCV slightly reduced Occasional target cells (20–30% Hb E)	SE Asia (up to 30% of population)
Haemoglobin C	CC Chronic haemolysis and large spleen Mild anaemia Reticulocytes increased Target cells are prominent	AC Normal Target cells	West Africa
Haemoglobin D**	DD Normal Hb level	AD Normal Hb level	NW India

*Individuals with Hb E commonly co-inherit thalassaemia.

**May be confused with Hb S on electrophoresis. Distinction is important for genetic counselling.

Q14 What other pathological mechanisms can contribute to the clinical signs and symptoms of sickle cell disease?

A Damage to the endothelium (lining of the blood vessels) occurs in sickle cell disease. The red cells containing haemoglobin S have an increased adhesiveness (stickiness) and this can cause blockage to normal blood flow in these vessels.

> **Key point**
> Decreased blood flow contributes significantly to the hypoxic organ damage.

Q15 What other clinical problems occur in patients with sickle cell disease?

A There are many clinical problems as a direct result of the abnormal haemoglobin in the red cells (Table 7.4).

Table 7.4 The main clinical problems in individuals with sickle cell disease

Problem	Reason
1 Stroke in young patients	Due to occlusion of the blood vessels.
2 Dactylitis in young children	Due to bone marrow necrosis in the hands and the feet. The blood supply to the marrow is reduced because of the sickle cells.
3 Severe infection	Splenic infarction because of the reduced blood supply caused by the sickle cells. Reduced splenic function increases the risk of infection with encapsulated bacteria, e.g. *Streptococcus pneumoniae.*
4 Pregnancy	Pre-eclampsia because of sickle cells in the placental blood supply. This may also cause abortion.
5 Avascular necrosis of the head of the femur	The blood supply is impaired because of the 'sickling' of the red cells.
6 Priapism	Painful erections in males due to 'sickling' and stagnation of blood in the penis.
7 Folate deficiency	Chronic haemolysis may lead to a further fall in Hb. Patients should take folate supplements routinely.
8 Gallstones	Chronic haemolysis increases the bilirubin turnover and may cause 'pigment' stones.

Q16 What else can be done to prevent these infectious complications?

A Pneumococcal vaccination and antibiotic prophylaxis (penicillin).

This will reduce the risk of lethal infection. In young patients, stem cell transplantation can be an option.

Recently, it has been shown that the drug hydroxyurea, an inhibitor of ribonucleotide reductase, can significantly increase the level of foetal haemoglobin (Hb F) in patients with sickle cell disease. This will reduce the number of painful crises.

> **Key point**
> Frequent blood transfusion in children will reduce the risk of stroke.

Q17 Can you now construct an algorithm to investigate an individual of African descent with anaemia and a history of blood transfusion?

A Yes.

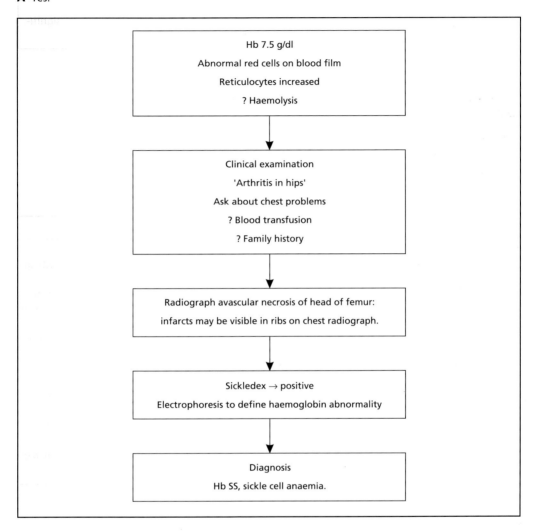

Ola made a slow recovery. His temperature returned to normal and his breathing and chest radiograph gradually improved and the need for narcotic analgesia decreased. He was discharged from hospital 4 weeks later and was asked to attend the haematology clinic. He was given hydroxyurea in an attempt to reduce the number of painful crises and to reduce the need for blood transfusion.

Suggested reading

Embury, S.H. & Vichinsky, E.P. (2000) Sickle cell disease. In: *Hematology. Basic Principles and Practice* (eds R. Hoffman, E.J. Benz, Jr, S.J. Shattil, B. Furie, H.J. Cohen, L.E. Silberstein & P. McGlave), 3rd edn, pp. 510–54. Churchill Livingstone, New York, USA.

Miller, S.T., Sleeper, L.A., Pegelow, C.H., *et al.* (2000) Prediction of adverse outcomes in children with sickle cell disease. *New England Journal of Medicine*, **342**, 83–9.

Wild, B.J. & Bain, B.J. (2001) Investigation of abnormal haemoglobins and thalassaemia. In: *Practical Haematology* (eds S.M. Lewis, B.J. Bain & I. Bates), 9th edn, pp. 231–68. Churchill Livingstone, London, UK

Rees, D.C., Olujohungbe, A.D., Parker, N.E., Stephens, A.D., Tellfer, P. & Wright, J. (2003) Guidelines for the management of the acute painful crisis in sickle cell disease. *British Journal of Haematology*, **120** (5), 744–52.

Sickle Cell Anemia, NHLBI. www.nhlbi.nih.gov/health/public/blood/sickle/sca_fact.htm

A young girl from Sardinia with thalassaemia

Luisa Corelli, a 19-year-old woman, has just moved to your locality from her native Sardinia. She tells you she has a history of thalassaemia and needs follow-up care.

Q1 **What steps should be taken to support the diagnosis?**

A A history and physical examination. Obtain full blood count (Table 8.1), blood film (Fig. 8.1) from the hospital in which the diagnosis was originally made and liver blood tests (see Table 8.4).

She says she commenced a chronic transfusion programme when she was aged 6. She requires red cell transfusion every 6–8 weeks. She has hy-

pothyroidism and takes thyroxine replacement. She has been told recently that her blood glucose is slightly elevated. She is also taking an ACE inhibitor for mild cardiac failure.

On examination she was small in stature and her skin had a bronze colour. Her spleen was enlarged and palpable 2 cm below her left costal margin.

Table 8.1 Full blood count at the time of diagnosis

	Patient's results	Normal range
Hb	5.2 g/dl	11.5–16.4 g/dl
MCV	59 fl	83–98 fl (μm^3)
WBC	4.2×10^9/l	$3.5–11.0 \times 10^9$/l (10^3/μl)
Platelets	389×10^9/l	$140–450 \times 10^9$/l (10^3/μl)
Reticulocyte count	480×10^9/l	$20–100 \times 10^9$/l (0.2–1.5%)

The differential white cell count was normal. The blood film (Fig. 8.1) showed hypochromic microcytic red cells, red cell fragments, nucleated red cells and polychromasia.

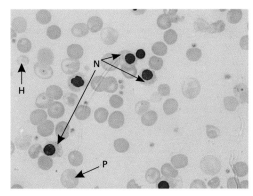

Figure 8.1 A blood film showing hypochromic microcytic red cells (H), nucleated red cells (N) and polychromasia (P).

A The bronze colour could be explained by iron deposition in the skin, but the blood film suggests a reduction in the amount of Hb in each red cell and evidence of haemolysis (polychromasia, nucleated red cells and an elevated reticulocyte count). The large spleen is due to a combination of haemolysis and extramedullary haemopoiesis.

A Iron deficiency, because it also presents with a low Hb and decreased MCH and MCV but it will not have the other red cell changes and it will have a low serum ferritin, whereas thalassaemia will have a normal or high serum ferritin. Examination of the blood film (Fig. 8.1) and serum ferritin estimation should distinguish between the two conditions.

A Thalassaemia is a quantitative disorder of globin chain synthesis. There are two main types, α or β thalassaemia, depending on which pair of globin chains is synthesized ineffectively. Normally, globin chain synthesis is balanced and haemoglobin A, the predominant form of haemoglobin, consists of two α and two β chains. Each newly synthesized chain will pair appropriately to form haemoglobin, which is soluble within the red cell. In the homozygous thalassaemic state unbalanced α or β globin chain synthesis causes accumulation of insoluble, unpaired chains which are toxic to the red cell precursors and mature red cells, inducing both ineffective erythropoiesis and a haemolytic anaemia. The β thalassaemias result from over 150 different mutations of the β globin genes, which decrease the production of β globin chains, either completely or partially. They are inherited as autosomal recessive genes in similar fashion to qualitative disorders of haemoglobin synthesis, e.g. Hb SS (see Case 7).

A Using haemoglobin electrophoresis to identify variant haemoglobins. This technique exposes proteins to a charge gradient and they are separated from each other by their size and charge. (Fig. 8.2).

Bands of Hb A$_2$ and Hb F only were seen.

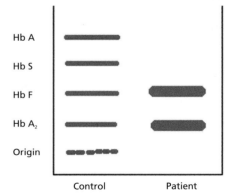

Figure 8.2 Hb electrophoresis showing the presence of Hb A$_2$, Hb F and the absence of Hb A.

A Each type of haemoglobin is composed of two different pairs of polypeptide chains (Table 8.2). The structure of haemoglobin changes during development. By the 12th week of gestation, embryonic haemoglobin is replaced by foetal haemoglobin, which is slowly replaced after birth by the adult haemoglobins Hb A and Hb A_2. In adults 96–98% of haemoglobin is haemoglobin A, which has two α chains and two β chains. Hb A has the structure of $\alpha_2\beta_2$ (two α chains and two β chains). The globin chains enfold a haem moiety consisting of a porphyrin ring complexed with a single iron atom. Each haem moiety can bind a single molecule of oxygen.

Table 8.2 The different types of Hb during development

Haemoglobin (Hb)	Globin chains	Period when normally present
A	$\alpha_2\beta_2$	Major Hb in adult life
A_2	$\alpha_2\delta_2$	Minor Hb in adult life
F	$\alpha_2\gamma_2$	Minor Hb in adult life, major Hb in foetal life with declining % during neonatal period
Gower 1/2	$\zeta_2\varepsilon_2 / \zeta_2\alpha_2$	Significant Hb during early intrauterine life
Portland 1/2	$\zeta_2\gamma_2 / \zeta_2\beta_2$	Significant Hb during early intrauterine life

A β thalassaemia major, because of the transfusion-dependent anaemia, splenomegaly and absence of Hb A on electrophoresis (β chains are necessary for the synthesis of Hb A).

A Heterozygotes for β thalassaemia (thalassaemia trait) are usually completely asymptomatic except in times of haemopoietic stress, for example during pregnancy. The blood count characteristically shows a normal or slightly reduced Hb, a reduction in the MCH and MCV and an elevated RBC count. The diagnosis depends upon the detection of an increased Hb A_2 %. Homozygotes develop anaemia in the first year of life. The excess α chains precipitate in the red cell precursors, leading to premature destruction. The bone marrow compensates by increasing the number of reticulocytes. This bone marrow expansion leads to changes in the skull and long bones.

A Iron deposition in the endocrine organs.

A Serum ferritin (Table 8.3).

Table 8.3 Serum ferritin results

	Patient's results	Normal range
Ferritin	3800 µg/l	20–300 µg/l (ng/ml)

Q11 Why might Luisa be at risk of iron deposition in her organs and what other organs might be involved?

A The major complication of thalassaemia is iron overload.

The excess iron becomes deposited in the tissues, particularly the heart and liver, which if untreated can lead to a cardiomyopathy or liver disease. The human body has no effective way of removing excess iron other than bleeding.

> **Key point**
> Each unit of red cells (250 ml) contains approximately 125 mg of iron.

Q12 What other abnormalities/deficiencies could contribute to her anaemia?

A Folate deficiency because of the chronic haemolysis.

All patients with significant degrees of thalassaemia should receive folate acid supplements on a daily basis indefinitely.

Q13 How can the abnormal facial and skull appearance be explained?

A Expansion of the marrow cavity to compensate for the severe anaemia (Fig. 8.3).

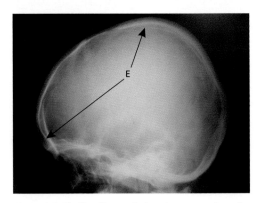

Figure 8.3 Skull radiograph showing expansion of the cranial bone marrow cavity due to ineffective haematopoiesis. It is also called hair on end appearance.

Q14 What other complications of blood transfusions can you anticipate?

A Transfusion transmitted viral infections are a major problem for thalassaemic patients who commenced their transfusion programme before blood donations were routinely tested for the viruses which cause hepatitis and AIDS. Chronic viral hepatitis and hepatic siderosis can act synergistically to promote chronic liver disease.

Her hepatitis B serology was normal and she was Anti-HCV (hepatitis C virus) positive, meaning she had been exposed to the hepatitis C virus. A subsequent test showed she was HCV RNA positive, demonstrating ongoing replication of the hepatitis C virus. Her HIV serology was negative.

Table 8.4 Liver blood tests (LBTs)

	Patient's results	Normal range
AST (SGOT)	47 IU/l	7–40 IU/l
Alkaline phosphatase	130 IU/l	40–120 IU/l
GGT	62 IU/l	10–55 IU/l
Random blood glucose	13.0 mmol/l	<11.1 mmol/l (<200 mg/ml)

Q15 In view of the above, what abnormalities of the LBTs would you expect (see Table 8.4)?

A Many patients with hepatitis C are asymptomatic and their blood tests relatively normal. Chronic hepatitis occurs in about 50–70% of those infected with hepatitis C. Among asymptomatic people with Anti-HCV, between 33% and 50% have evidence of inflammation on liver biopsy.

Q16 What are the principles of treatment?

A Red cell transfusion to relieve anaemia, iron chelation and consideration of the possibility of allogeneic stem cell transplantation if a suitable donor is available.

A Phlebotomy is the most efficient and least toxic way to remove excess iron; however, it is not applicable in someone like Luisa who is anaemic. The most effective method of iron chelation is desferrioxamine, which binds iron and promotes its excretion in the urine. It has to be administered by continuous subcutaneous infusion for 8 to 12 hours daily (Fig. 8.4).

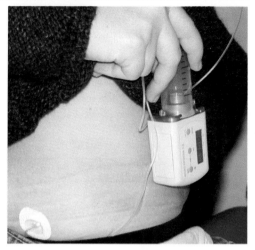

Figure 8.4 Iron chelation therapy being administered via an infusion pump.

Luisa has been prescribed desferrioxamine 5 nights per week for 12 hours. She admits that over the last few years she has been missing some of the doses as it interferes with her lifestyle.

> **Key point**
> Because of difficulties with compliance, oral iron chelators are currently being evaluated.

Three months later Luisa attends the surgery acutely unwell. She has a 2-day history of right upper quadrant colicky abdominal pain and nausea. She has a tachycardia of 120 beats/min. She has a temperature of 38.5°C and is acutely tender in the right upper quadrant with guarding and localized rebound tenderness.

Q18 What might explain these symptoms and signs?

A Acute cholecystitis (inflammation of the gall-bladder).

Q19 Why should a patient of her age develop cholecystitis?

A Patients with chronic haemolytic anaemia (as part of her thalassemia syndrome) are more likely to have pigment gallstones. Acute inflammation of the gall-bladder usually follows obstruction of the cystic duct by a stone.

The presence of increased amounts of insoluble bilirubin in bile results in the precipitation of the bilirubin which aggregates and forms pigment stones.

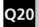

Q20 Can you now construct an algorithm for a patient with severe microcytic hypochromic anaemia?

A Yes.

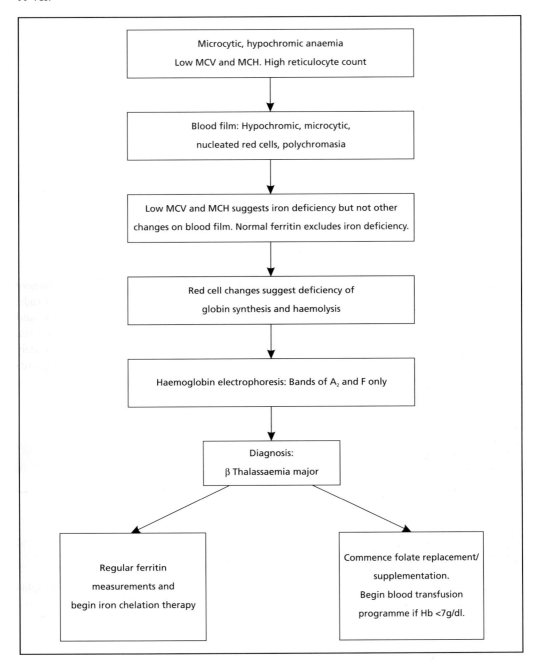

OUTCOME

Luisa was admitted to hospital where the diagnosis of acute cholecystitis was confirmed. An abdominal ultrasound confirmed the presence of stones. She was treated with intravenous antibiotics for 3 days; however, she remained very ill. A laparotomy and cholecystectomy were performed. Post-operatively, she developed acute heart failure, which was felt to be secondary to a cardiomyopathy from her iron overload. She was treated with diuretics but unfortunately continued to deteriorate. She died in the intensive care unit 48 hours after her surgery.

Suggested reading

Lukens, J.H. (1999) The thalassaemias and related disorders: quantitative disorders of haemoglobin synthesis. In: *Wintrobe's Clinical Hematology* (eds G.R. Lee, J. Foerster, J. Lukens, F. Paraskevas, J.P. Greer & G.M. Rodgers), 10th edn, Vol. 1, Chapter 53, pp. 1405–1448. Williams and Wilkins, Baltimore, USA.

Olivieri, N.F. (1999) The ß-thalassemias. *New England Journal of Medicine*, **341**, 99–109.

Hoffbrand, A.V., Pettit, J.E. & Moss, P.A.H. (2001) *Essential Haematology*, 4th edn. Blackwell Science, Oxford. See Chapter 6: Genetic disorders of haemoglobin.

Weatherall, D.J. & Clegg, J.B. (2001) *The Thalassaemia Syndromes*, 4th edn. Blackwell Science, Oxford.

Wild, V.J. & Bain, B.J. (2001) Investigation of abnormal haemoglobins and thalassaemia. In: *Practical Haematology* (eds S.M. Lewis, B.J. Bain & I. Bates), 9th edn, Chapter 12, pp. 231–268. Churchill Livingstone, London, UK.

A young boy with a sore throat and bleeding gums

A mother brought her 17-year-old boy to the family doctor because he had a sore throat, bleeding from his gums and a rash on his ankles. He had vomited on three occasions the evening before and had developed two red eyes. He was a schoolboy and denied cigarette smoking, alcohol intake or using illicit substances. He had been perfectly well until 3 weeks before.

The doctor noted a red appearance in his throat, bilateral sub-conjunctival haemorrhages and some petechiae on his legs. The doctor was unable to palpate any lymph nodes or enlargement of the liver or spleen. His temperature was elevated at 38°C. He looked pale.

Q1 | **How can the physical findings be linked?**

A A sore throat suggests infection and pallor suggests anaemia. The presence of sub-conjunctival bleeding and petechiae would suggest a low platelet count. Bleeding into joints or muscles, in contrast, indicates a coagulopathy.

The bone marrow (the factory which produces blood) may not be functioning properly and the production of red cells and platelets becomes deficient. The findings could also be explained by premature destruction of red cells and platelets.

Q2 | **What should be done next?**

A Arrange for the patient to be seen immediately by a haematologist or otherwise attend the Accident and Emergency Department at the nearest hospital.

Q3 | **What therapeutic approach should be taken to treat his fever?**

A In adults it is rarely necessary to treat a fever. In young children, however, high fevers can cause febrile convulsions and should be treated.

A Paracetamol. Aspirin should not be given to a patient with a low platelet count.

> **Key point**
> Aspirin interferes with platelet function (it does not alter platelet numbers) through its inhibition of cyclooxygenase and could initiate bleeding (especially if the platelet count is low.

A They can cause bleeding into the muscle (haematoma) in the presence of a low platelet count and should not be used until the platelet count has been measured.

The patient arrived at the Accident and Emergency Department of the hospital 1 hour later, with a letter from the family doctor.

A Take a detailed medical history, asking about any recent travel, medications and use of recreational drugs or possible exposure to infection with viruses, including HIV. A history of jaundice should be specifically enquired about.

As stated to the family doctor, there were no medications. Travel and use of recreational drugs or exposure to possible HIV infection were denied.

A The presence of the patient's mother might inhibit the patient from admitting to the use of recreational drugs or exposure to HIV infection.

Following the history, the doctor examined the patient and confirmed the findings of the family doctor without additional abnormalities (Figs 9.1 and 9.2).

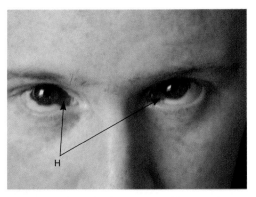

Figure 9.1 Bilateral sub-conjunctival haemorrhages (H).

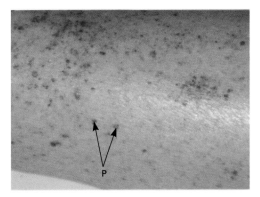

Figure 9.2 A petechial rash (P) on his leg.

Q8   What should the doctor do next?

A A blood count (Table 9.1), coagulation screen, liver, renal and bone profile, urinalysis, blood pressure and chest radiograph.

There was a trace of haemolysed blood in the urine.

Table 9.1 Blood test results

	Patient's results	Normal range (male)
Hb	8.9 g/dl	13.5–18.0 g/dl
Red cell count	3.0×10^{12}/l	$4.60–5.70 \times 10^{12}$/l (10^6/µl)
MCV	103 fl	83–99 fl (µm³)
WBC	2.2×10^9/l	$4.0–11.0 \times 10^9$/l (10^3/µl)
Platelets	18×10^9/l	$140–450 \times 10^9$/l (10^3/µl)
Neutrophils	0.2×10^9/l	$2.0–7.5 \times 10^9$/l (10^3/µl)
Lymphocytes	2.3×10^9/l	$1.5–3.5 \times 10^9$/l (10^3/µl)
Reticulocytes	24×10^9/l	$20–100 \times 10^9$/l (0.2–1.5%)

Q9   How can these blood findings be interpreted?

A A decrease in the Hb, neutrophil and platelet count is known as 'pancytopenia'.

The fact that the red cells are larger than normal (elevated MCV) suggests a defect in the maturation of the red cells in the bone marrow or an increase in the number of young circulating red cells (known as reticulocytes). However, a low reticulocyte count suggests a difficulty in manufacturing red cells. The reduced neutrophil and platelet count suggests that the production problem might also be affecting these cells.

In view of the elevated MCV (macrocytosis), blood should be sent for an estimation of serum vitamin B_{12} and red cell folate.

A The low platelet count explains the rash on the patient's legs and the sub-conjunctival bleeding.

> **Key point**
> Bleeding will occur after minor trauma if the platelet count is below $50 \times 10^9/l$. Bleeding will occur spontaneously if the platelet count goes below $10 \times 10^9/l$.

The raised intracranial pressure (as a result of the vomiting) precipitated the boy's sub-conjunctival bleeding. Sub-conjunctival bleeding is of no danger to the patient's vision. It alerts us to the presence of a low platelet count and unless prompt corrective action is taken quickly, there is a risk of intracranial bleeding. The retina should be examined immediately for fresh haemorrhages. Retinal haemorrhages can interfere with vision, especially if they occur in the area of the macula. It is important to measure the blood pressure when the platelet count is low. The presence of an elevated systolic blood pressure significantly increases the risk of serious retinal or intracranial bleeding and should be treated as an emergency. In this case, the blood pressure was within normal limits. The rash on the legs is due to bleeding into the skin, known as purpura, which is due to the low platelet count. Purpura can be confluent, in which case, it is called a bruise or ecchymosis or it can be punctate and appear as small red dots like pinpoints. These dots are known as petechiae. The reason that this type of bleeding occurs predominantly in the legs is simply because when we are walking there is increased hydrostatic pressure in the small blood vessels of the skin.

The doctor examined the patient's retina and there were no retinal haemorrhages. The trace of blood in his urine was insignificant and can occur with a low platelet count. The coagulation, biochemical screens and chest radiograph were normal.

A The coagulation screen is not influenced by the platelet count.

> **Key point**
> The role of the patient's platelet count is overridden by the addition of a substitute for the platelet phospholipid in the prothrombin time, PT, and the activated partial thromboplastin time, APTT.

A Admit the patient to hospital immediately and arrange a bone marrow aspirate and biopsy.

A There is no need to give platelets prior to the aspiration and biopsy of marrow from the posterior iliac crest. Firm digital pressure should be applied for 5 minutes or until the bleeding stops. A firm pressure dressing should then be applied and inspected 30 minutes later for bleeding (Figs 9.3 and 9.4).

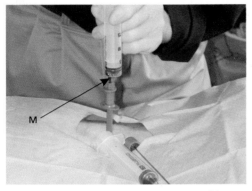

Figure 9.3 Bone marrow (M) being aspirated from the posterior iliac crest.

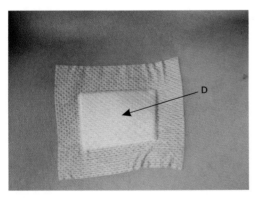

Figure 9.4 A pressure dressing (D) applied to the aspirate site.

Pressure dressings should be small and tightly applied. Large dressings will only obscure bleeding and rarely exert adequate pressure.

The bone marrow aspirate was reported as 'hypoplastic', with a few marrow cells present but no abnormal cells were seen. No megaloblastic features were present to suggest a deficiency of vitamin B_{12} or folic acid. The marrow biopsy also revealed severe hypoplasia and again no abnormal cells were seen.

The vitamin B_{12} and folate levels were normal. Vitamin B_{12} deficiency would be extremely rare in a patient of this age. Folate deficiency could be present secondary to coeliac disease. In folate or B_{12} deficiency causing a pancytopenia, the biochemical screen would be abnormal with elevated levels of bilirubin and lactic dehydrogenase indicating ineffective erythropoiesis (premature destruction of haemopoietic cells in the marrow).

The marrow aspirate and biopsy complement each other. The aspirate allows us to examine individual cells in detail and the biopsy allows us to assess the marrow architecture. The biopsy (Figs 9.5 and 9.6) is especially useful in assessing the 'cellularity' of the marrow and the presence of non-haemopoietic cells such as metastatic cancer.

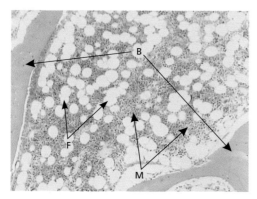

Figure 9.5 A normal marrow biopsy. Marrow cells (M) are seen between the fat spaces (F). Bony trebeculae (B) are pink.

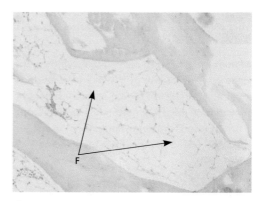

Figure 9.6 A marrow biopsy from a patient with severe aplastic anaemia. Most of the normal marrow is replaced by fat spaces (F).

Q14 How might the blood and bone marrow test results be linked to the clinical findings?

A Since the marrow biopsy reveals a severe reduction in the number of marrow cells present and there is no evidence of abnormal cells the diagnosis is 'aplastic anaemia'.

Aplastic anaemia is a rare condition in which the marrow elements are severely reduced in the absence of abnormal cells. Although drugs and viral infections rarely precede the onset of aplastic anaemia, the aetiology is unknown in the majority of cases (Table 9.2).

There is a large amount of laboratory and clinical evidence to suggest that the pathogenesis of aplastic anaemia is autoimmune in most cases.

Table 9.2 Some drugs and viruses linked to aplastic anaemia

Drugs linked to aplastic anaemia	Viruses linked to aplastic anaemia
Chloramphenicol	Epstein–Barr virus
Cotrimoxazole	Hepatitis B virus
Chloroquin	HIV virus
Anti-inflammatories	
Gold salts	
Penicillamine	
Carbimazole	
Phenothiazines	
Carbamazepine	
Phenytoin	

In clinical practice you rarely find any cause for aplastic anaemia. A virus is rarely incriminated as a causal agent even if liver blood tests suggest a recent viral infection.

> **Key point**
> The spleen is not enlarged in patients with aplastic anaemia. If the spleen is enlarged another explanation for the pancytopenia should be sought.

What are the principles of treatment?

A Patients rarely recover and in the severe forms of the disease the majority of patients will die from infection or bleeding within a few months unless the underlying defect is corrected. The most effective treatment for severe aplastic anaemia is sibling (brother or sister) stem cell transplantation.

Q16 **What alternative treatment is available if a family donor is not found?**

A Treatment with powerful immunosuppressive agents (anti-thymocyte globulin and cyclosporine without giving stem cells) is frequently effective (up to 70%).

Q17 **Which inherited conditions manifest as aplastic anaemia?**

A The most common of these rare conditions is Fanconi anaemia.

This disorder is associated with two genetic abnormalities on chromosome 9 and 16, which leads to defective DNA repair. Clinically, there are often many abnormalities including short stature, pigmentation, skeletal and renal abnormalities, and aplastic anaemia. Those affected have an increased risk of developing acute myeloid leukaemia and solid tumours.

A Yes.

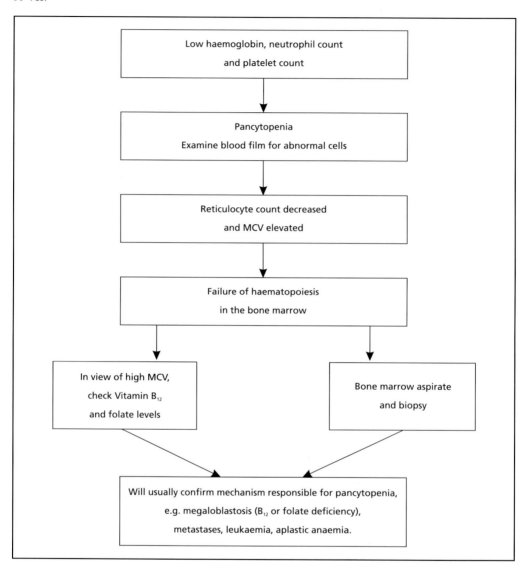

OUTCOME

The patient had a HLA compatible sister and he received a bone marrow transplant within 1 month of his diagnosis. His transplant was uncomplicated and he is now a 4th year medical student.

Bone marrow transplantation successfully cures >70% of young adults with aplastic anaemia if a compatible family donor is available.

Suggested reading

Schrezenmeier, H. & Bacigalupo, A. (1999) *Aplastic Anaemia. Pathophysiology and Treatment.* Cambridge University Press, Cambridge.

(2000) Acquired aplastic anemias. *Seminars in Haematology*, **37**, 1.

Young, N.S. (2000) Aplastic anemia. In: *Hematology. Basic Principles and Practice* (eds R. Hoffman, E.J. Benz, Jr, S.J. Shattil, B. Furie, H.J. Cohen, L.E. Silberstein & P. McGlave), 3rd edn, pp. 297–331. Churchill Livingstone, New York, USA.

Young, N.S. & Beris, P. (2001) Aplastic anemia. In: *Essential Haematology* (eds A.V. Hoffbrand, J.E. Pettit & P.A.H. Moss), 4th edn, pp. 91–7. Blackwell Science, Oxford.

Marsh, J.C.W., Ball, S.E., Darbyshire, P. *et al.* (2003) Guidelines for the diagnosis and management of aplastic anaemia. *British Journal of Haematology*, **123**, 782–801.

A football player who was dropped from the team

John, a 35-year-old pharmaceutical hospital specialist was 'dropped' from the rugby team. He admitted to the coach that he had been feeling unusually tired for the last 6 months and had occasional episodes of sweating, especially at night. He went to his family doctor.

The only additional symptom that John mentioned was occasional discomfort in his left upper abdomen. He did not smoke and he consumed 20 units of alcohol weekly. He had never been in hospital, was taking no medication and denied the use of recreational drugs.

Q1 What might be causing his symptoms?

A Fatigue could be caused by anaemia or depression, and 'sweating' could be a manifestation of infection.

Q2 How is sweating evaluated?

A Ask: 'Did you have to change your bed clothes because of the night sweat?'

Anxiety, hyperthyroidism, infections (e.g. tuberculosis) and some haematological malignancies (e.g. non-Hodgkin's lymphoma, chronic myeloid leukaemia) can cause sweating. A travel history should be taken since infections (such as malaria), not commonly seen in Europe, can present in this way. A full physical examination should be undertaken.

Q3 What should be done next?

A A full physical examination.

The man appeared healthy. There was no evidence of weight loss and the only abnormal finding was an enlarged spleen, palpable 4 cm below the left costal margin on quiet inspiration. There was no lymphadenopathy and his chest was clinically clear.

A The spleen lies between the 9th and 11th ribs posteriorly. It is not normally palpable. Occasionally in a very thin individual you may be able to palpate the tip of the spleen on deep inspiration.

In this case the spleen was easily palpable on quiet inspiration and, therefore, is significantly enlarged (Fig. 10.1).

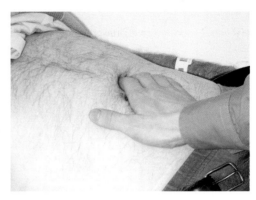

Figure 10.1 Palpation of a large spleen extending below the left lower ribs.

Q5   **What diseases might cause an enlarged spleen in an otherwise healthy looking young man?**

A A palpable spleen in an otherwise healthy looking young man suggests either a haematological disorder or an increase in blood flow through the spleen, causing it to enlarge (e.g. portal hypertension). In tropical areas infections such as malaria and schistosomiasis may cause a large spleen.

Q6   **How reliable is physical examination in assessing spleen size?**

A It is reliable for an experienced examiner. However, in obese individuals it may be very difficult to feel a slightly enlarged spleen.

Q7   What investigation will define the size of the spleen?

A Ultrasound examination of the abdomen is a reliable, non-invasive, inexpensive test (Fig. 10.2).

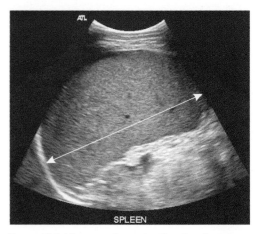

Figure 10.2 Ultrasound examination showing an enlarged spleen (the dark grey area outlined by the arrow) measuring 13.8 cm (normal is 11–12 cm).

Q8   What investigations might help to find the cause of the enlarged spleen?

A A full blood count, blood film, reticulocyte count and a biochemical screen (Tables 10.1 and 10.2).

Table 10.1 Full blood and reticulocyte count

	Patient's results	Normal range (male)
Hb	14.0 g/dl	13.5–18.0 g/dl
WBC	55.0 × 10⁹/l	4.0–11.0 × 10⁹/l (10³/µl)
Platelets	600 × 10⁹/l	140–450 × 10⁹/l (10³/µl)
Reticulocyte count	64.0 × 10⁹/l	20–100 × 10⁹/l (0.2–1.5%)

Table 10.2 Lactic dehydrogenase and urate (uric acid) results

	Patient's results	Normal range
Lactic dehydrogenase (LDH)	850 IU/l	230–450 IU/l
Urate (uric acid)	600 µmol/l	150–470 µmol/l (3–8 mg/dl)

There was a marked increase in the white cell count. White cell precursors including meta-myelocytes, myelocytes and promyelocytes were present (Fig. 10.3).

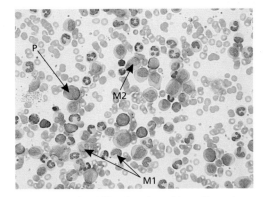

Figure 10.3 Blood film showing white cell precursors, metamyelocytes (M1), myelocytes (M2) and promyelocytes (P).

Q9 What do these blood results indicate?

A The Hb is normal and the white cell count is elevated. White cell precursors are present. These cells are normally found in the bone marrow and not in the peripheral blood. The platelet count is also elevated. This suggests that the bone marrow is overactive and releasing white cells and platelets prematurely into the circulation. The results of these tests therefore suggest a severe disturbance of the bone marrow, not an infectious disease.

Q10 What should be done next?

A He should be referred to a haematologist because he has a significant haematological disorder.

The patient received an appointment to see a haematologist 2 days later. He was advised not to play rugby and to avoid strenuous exercise.

Q11 Why was this advice given?

A It is possible to rupture an enlarged spleen following trauma. This could lead to life-threatening intra-abdominal bleeding.

He was interviewed and examined by the haematologist, who repeated the blood count and blood film and received the results of the biochemical screen and ultrasound examination.

Q12 How would the haematologist interpret the blood findings?

A The most likely diagnosis in a young man with a large spleen and this blood picture is chronic myeloid leukaemia (CML). It is possible in severe infections or when there are marrow metastases to have an elevated white cell count and to see white cell and red cell precursors in the blood (a leucoerythroblastic blood picture). There are a number of possible causes of a large spleen, such as chronic infection with malaria, liver disease with portal hypertension, non-Hodgkin's lymphomas and chronic lymphocytic leukaemia, but none of these conditions will have the peripheral blood findings as described in this patient.

Q13 How are the biochemical results explained?

A The elevated LDH (see Table 10.2) reflects cell death and is non-specific. It could be elevated following myocardial infarction, liver damage or premature death of blood cells. In this case it reflects death of white blood cells. Similarly, the elevated uric acid level in the plasma reflects increased cell turnover.

Q14 What should be done next?

A A bone marrow examination was arranged, since a serious haematological disorder was suspected.

Q15 From which site was the bone marrow aspirated?

A The posterior iliac crest. It is the least painful site for the patient and almost completely without hazard. Care should be taken to make sure that adequate local analgesia is given and that there is no bleeding after the procedure.

Q16 What investigations would the haematologist request on the sample of bone marrow?

A Slides for microscopic examination. A sample should be also sent to the genetics department for a karyotypic (cytogenetic) analysis.

Q17 How does the bone marrow aspirate help to confirm the suspected diagnosis?

A The slides revealed a very cellular specimen with increased numbers of white blood cell and platelet precursors (megakaryocytes), suggesting increased marrow activity or reduced cell death (apoptosis).

A A biopsy of the bone marrow (Figs 10.4 and 10.5), also from the posterior iliac crest, will yield complementary information.

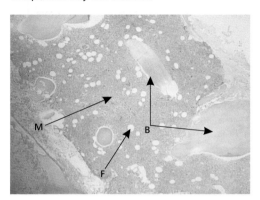

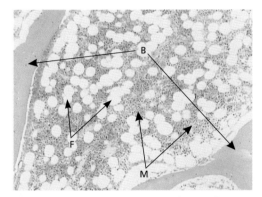

Figure 10.4 A bone marrow biopsy showing a hypercellular marrow (M). Bony trabeculae (B) are shown in pink. Fat spaces (F) are reduced.

Figure 10.5 A normal bone marrow biopsy showing bone marrow cells (M), bony trabeculae (B) and fat spaces (F).

Q19 How should the patient be managed?

A The probable diagnosis should be explained to the patient. If he has a partner she should be invited, with the patient's permission, to come back in a few days to discuss the result of the outstanding tests. The patient should be assured that there is no immediate danger, but be advised to remain off work and refrain from contact sports until the diagnosis is clarified.

Q20 What medications would the haematologist prescribe?

A Allopurinol, a competitive inhibitor of xanthine oxidase. This drug will reduce the level of urate (uric acid) in the plasma and decrease the risk of gout and renal damage.

The patient and his partner were given the results 3 days later.

The cytogenetic analysis revealed a normal number of chromosomes but a small chromosome number 22 (Fig. 10.6). This was due to a translocation of a portion of chromosome 9 to chromosome 22 and a reciprocal (reverse) transfer of a portion of chromosome from chromosome 22 to chromosome 9 (Fig. 10.7).

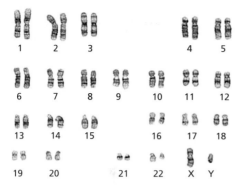

Figure 10.6 The abnormally small chromosome 22, the 'Philadelphia' chromosome.

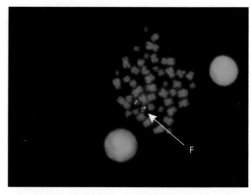

Figure 10.7 FISH analysis (fluorescent in situ hybridization) of bone marrow cells showing fusion of BCR/ABL (F).

Q21 Why is this small chromosome 22 called the 'Philadelphia' chromosome and what is its significance?

A The small, abnormal chromosome 22 was first described by two scientists in patients with CML in Philadelphia.

This translocation was the first non-random, reproducible chromosomal abnormality to be described in a human cancer. It is always present in the bone marrow cells of patients with CML. It is very significant in our understanding of the pathogenesis of CML. When portions of different chromosomes come together the production of an abnormal gene product (protein) occurs. In the case of CML the abnormal gene product influences cell division and programmed cell death (apoptosis). The fusion gene on chromosome 22 is called BCR/ABL (Fig. 10.8).

Key point

The abnormal chromosome found in CML causes the malignant phenotype, i.e. makes the cells behave in a cancerous way. In very recent times this knowledge has stimulated the development of drugs which specifically inhibit these abnormalities and induce apoptosis of the leukaemia cells.

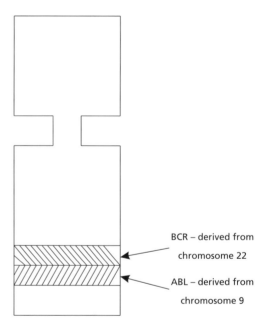

BCR – derived from chromosome 22

ABL – derived from chromosome 9

Figure 10.8 'Philadelphia' chromosome t(9:22), showing the two chromosomal fragments together on chromosome 22 that result in the synthesis of a protein, which causes the leukaemia cells to behave in a malignant way.

A Reassure both of them that there is no immediate danger and that all his symptoms should disappear following 3–4 weeks of treatment.

Q23 What is the long-term outlook for the patient?

A The only definitive treatment is a stem cell transplant from a HLA compatible sibling. As this patient has no siblings he will be treated medically.

A search for a HLA compatible volunteer donor should be carried out (there are over 6 million donors on the international panel). If a suitable donor is found, consideration should be given to a stem cell transplant, depending on his response to medical treatment.

Q24 Can you construct an algorithm for investigation of a patient with a high white cell count and a large spleen?

A Yes.

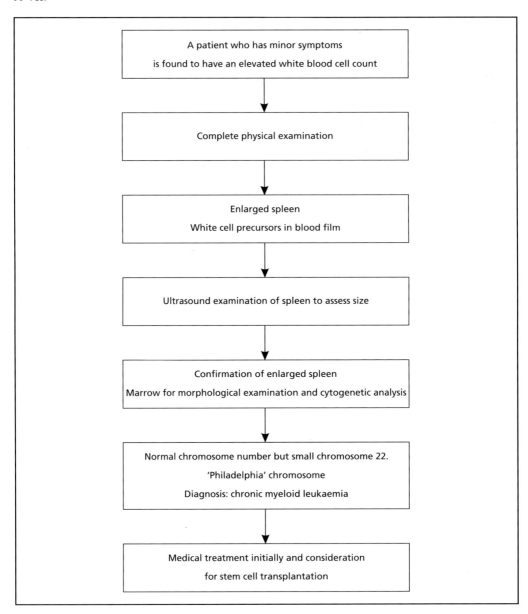

A patient who has minor symptoms
is found to have an elevated white blood cell count

↓

Complete physical examination

↓

Enlarged spleen
White cell precursors in blood film

↓

Ultrasound examination of spleen to assess size

↓

Confirmation of enlarged spleen
Marrow for morphological examination and cytogenetic analysis

↓

Normal chromosome number but small chromosome 22.
'Philadelphia' chromosome
Diagnosis: chronic myeloid leukaemia

↓

Medical treatment initially and consideration
for stem cell transplantation

OUTCOME

Imatinib mesylate, a new agent capable of inducing apoptosis in the leukaemia cells, was prescribed. He returned to work in a few days and was able to resume a normal life.

He is seen in the haematology clinic at monthly intervals.

Suggested reading

Sawyers, C.L. (2001) Mechanisms of leukemogenesis. In: *The Molecular Basis of Blood Diseases* (eds G. Stamatoyannopoulos, P.W. Majerus, P.M. Perlmutter & H. Varmus), 3rd edn, pp. 832–60. WB Saunders Company, Philadelphia, USA.

Sawyers, C.S. (1999) Chronic myeloid leukemia. *New England Journal of Medicine*, **340**, 1330–40.

Enright, H. & McGlave, P. (2000) Chronic myelogenous leukemia. In: *Hematology. Basic Principles and Practice* (eds R. Hoffman, E.J. Benz, Jr, S.J. Shattil, B. Furie, H.J. Cohen, L.E. Silberstein & P. McGlave), 3rd edn, pp. 1155–71. Churchill Livingstone, New York, USA.

(2001) Targeting the BCR-ABL tyrosine kinase on chronic myeloid leukemia (editorial). *New England Journal of Medicine*, **344** (14), 1084–6.

Carella, A.M., Daley, G.Q., Eaves, C.J., Goldmanand, J.M. & Hehlmann, R. (eds) (2001) *Chronic Myeloid Leukaemia. Biology and Treatment*. Martin Dunitz, London, UK.

A middle-aged man who cannot button his shirt collar

John is a 62-year-old Caucasian man who noticed a decrease in his energy over the last 2 weeks and a difficulty in buttoning his shirt collar. He had always been fit and energetic. He is a non-smoker and drinks only an occasional glass of wine at the weekend. He plays golf one afternoon per week.

Q1 What could cause his symptoms?

A The causes of a neck swelling that would make buttoning a collar difficult are quite limited. The swelling could be due to (i) an enlarged thyroid gland, (ii) enlarged lymph nodes, (iii) a mass not related to any local anatomical structure, e.g. metastases from a cancer elsewhere, (iv) obstruction of the superior vena cava, usually due to a tumour in the anterior mediastinum, or (v) inflammatory/infectious lesions in the mouth, throat or anywhere in the head and neck region.

Q2 What should be done next?

A Take a full history.

Q3 What are the important issues when taking the history?

A The duration the symptoms have been present. Ask specific questions and link them to an event in his personal life or a public event. Ask about the severity of his fatigue. Has it interfered with his golf? Is the swelling in his neck painful and has it increased in size? When enquiring about night sweats ask if the patient changes his/her bed clothes or night attire.

John had been at an important dinner in his golf club 4 months ago and had difficulty then with buttoning his shirt and tying his bow tie. For the past 2–3 months he played only 9 instead of 18 holes of golf and noted night sweats.

The swelling has never been painful and he thinks that it is increasing in size.

Obstruction of the superior vena cava would usually be accompanied by a feeling of 'fullness' in the head and by a dusky-blue appearance. A family history of thyroid disease is important as it may occur in more than one family member. Viral infections, such as infectious mononucleosis, can cause transient lymph node enlargement but would be very uncommon in a patient of this age. Other symptoms such as weight loss and night sweats commonly occur in diseases such as Hodgkin's disease, non-Hodgkin's lymphoma and chronic lymphocytic leukaemia.

There was no family history of thyroid disease. John had never been ill before, apart from a fractured clavicle as a teenager. He has been married for 35 years and has two children 33 and 31 years of age who are both in good health.

Q4 What should be done next?

A A physical examination.

The patient appeared well. His temperature was 37°C, blood pressure 125/75 mmHg. His mouth and throat appeared normal. He had enlarged lymph nodes in his cervical, submandibular and supraclavicular regions (3 × 2 cm) (Fig. 11.1). They were non-tender, firm and fixed. The overlying skin appeared normal. The nodes in his axillae and groin were also enlarged (3 × 3 cm). His spleen was palpable 5 cm below the left lower ribs.

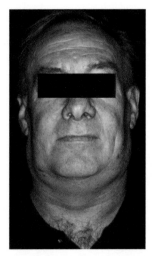

Figure 11.1 Enlarged lymph nodes in the neck.

Q5 What could be causing his symptoms and signs?

A Multiple enlarged lymph nodes, splenomegaly and fatigue are most likely due to a haematological malignancy.

A A full blood count (Table 11.1), blood film (Fig. 11.2), biochemical screen, a chest radiograph and computed tomography scan (CT) of the thorax and abdomen.

Table 11.1 Full blood count and blood film

	Patient's results	Normal range
Hb	14.2 g/dl	13.5–18.0 g/dl
WBC	55.0 × 10^9/l	4.0–11.00 × 10^9/l (10^3/μl)
Platelets	230 × 10^9/l	140–450 × 10^9/l (10^3/μl)
Neutrophils	5.5 × 10^9/l	2.0–7.5 × 10^9/l (10^3/μl)
Lymphocytes	49.5 × 10^9/l	1.5–3.5 × 10^9/l (10^3/μl)

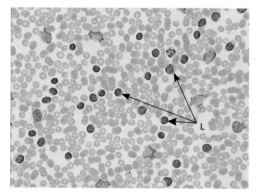

Figure 11.2 Blood film, showing a predominance of lymphocytes in the blood (L).

A He should be told that the diagnosis is not clear but there is a significant possibility that he has a serious blood disease. He could continue to work but should return, with his wife, for further discussion when the test results become available.

A The lymphocyte count is elevated, indicating an increased marrow output of lymphocytes.

The haemoglobin and platelet count are normal, therefore marrow function has been preserved.

In view of these findings John should be referred to a haematologist.

A Flow cytometry of the peripheral blood.

The lymphocyte population was made up almost entirely of B cells (normally T cells predominate in the blood). The B-lymphocytes were 'clonal', i.e. they expressed immunoglobulins on their cell surface with a single light chain only, κ or λ.

> **Key point**
> CLL is the most frequent leukaemia in the Western hemisphere. Although it usually occurs in the elderly (median age at presentation is 65 years), about 20% of patients are less than 60 years at the time of presentation. It occurs more frequently in men than in women.

Q10 **What could be the possible diagnosis?**

A Chronic lymphocytic leukaemia (CLL).

Q11 **Why is chronic lymphocytic leukaemia the most likely diagnosis?**

A The combination of a raised lymphocyte count, which were clonal, enlarged lymph nodes and spleen in a male patient aged 62 years are all typical findings in CLL.

> **Key point**
> There is an increased risk of CLL in first-degree relatives of patients with CLL.

The biochemical screen was normal. A CT scan of the thorax (Fig. 11.4) and abdomen (Fig. 11.5) showed enlarged lymph nodes, liver and spleen.

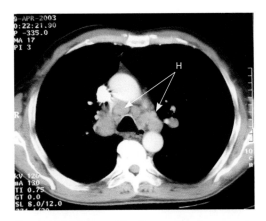

Figure 11.4 CT scan of the thorax, showing multiple enlarged mediastinal lymph nodes (H).

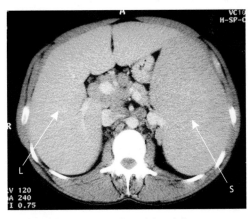

Figure 11.5 CT examination of the abdomen, showing a large liver (L) and spleen (S).

Q12 What should the haematologist do next?

A Interview the patient and repeat the history and physical examination. Carry out a bone marrow aspirate and biopsy (optional) (Fig. 11.3).

The physical findings were confirmed and a detailed history revealed that the patient thought that an elderly uncle had died from some form of leukaemia.

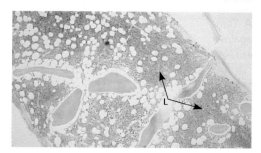

Figure 11.3 Bone marrow biopsy, showing a predominance of lymphocytes (L).

Q13 What further investigations should be carried out?

A The serum immunoglobulins (Table 11.2).

The cancer cells in CLL (as in most malignancies) are non-functional. Therefore, the level of immunoglobulins in the patient's serum is decreased (hypogammaglobulinaemia).

Table 11.2 Patient's immunoglobulin levels

	Patient's results	Normal range
IgG	3.0 g/l (300 mg/dl)	6.26–14.96 g/l (700–1450 mg/dl)
IgA	0.17 g/l (17 mg/dl)	0.62–2.90 g/l (70–370 mg/dl)
IgM	0.13 g/l (13 mg/dl)	0.47–1.82 g/l (30–210 mg/dl)

Q14 What infections occur in patients with hypogammaglobulinaemia?

A These patients are prone to respiratory infections with gram-positive encapsulated bacteria (Fig. 11.6).

> **Key point**
> Opsonization is a process where immunoglobulins coat bacteria with 'complement' sequences, leading to phagocytosis. This process is severely compromised in patients with CLL and hypogammaglobulinaemia.

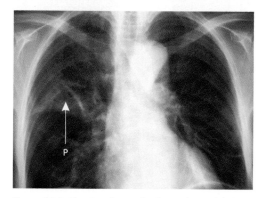

Figure 11.6 Chest radiograph of a patient with CLL with pneumonia.

Q15 What measures can be considered for patients with hypogammaglobulinaemia?

A These patients should receive vaccination against pneumococcus and haemophilus influenzae.

Q16 Why should patients with CLL and hypogammaglobulinaemia be vaccinated against the above infectious agents?

A The impairment of immunoglobulin (antibody synthesis) is not total and some antibody is made which clinically offers some protection from infection.

Q17 What measures can reduce the risk of recurring chest infections?

A Stop smoking. If recurrent infections are a problem, replacement therapy with human pooled immunoglobulins should be commenced.

Q18 What are the dangers of giving blood products manufactured from many litres of human plasma?

A There is a risk of transmitting HIV, hepatitis B or C, unknown viruses or prions.

> **Key point**
> The risk is minimal with careful screening of the donors, meticulous testing of the plasma products and steps taken in the manufacturing process to eliminate viruses.

A Infections with herpes viruses causing 'cold sores' or herpes zoster (Fig. 11.7).

> **Key point**
> In spite of hypogammaglobulinaemia, patients with CLL may experience severe autoimmune haemolytic anaemia.

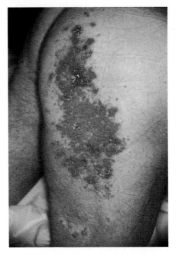

Figure 11.7 Herpes zoster infection affecting sciatic nerve distribution in a patient with CLL and hypogammaglobulinaemia.

Q20 What are the principles of treatment of patients with CLL?

A Not all patients require treatment. Treatment is considered when there is evidence of disease progression. Symptoms such as night sweats, weight loss and fatigue, extensive lymph node enlargement, anaemia or a low platelet count are all indications for treatment. More recently, combinations of chemotherapeutic agents and antibodies against CLL cells are being investigated. In younger patients the role of stem cell transplantation is being explored.

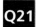 **Q21** Can you construct an algorithm to help you to investigate a middle-aged man or woman with enlarged lymph nodes in his/her neck?

A Yes.

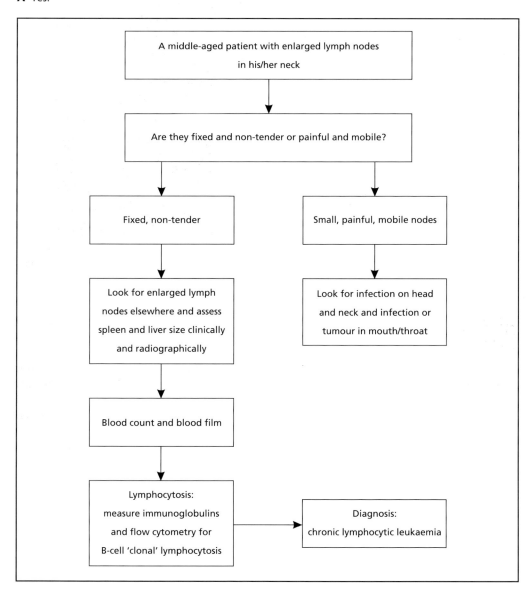

A middle-aged patient with enlarged lymph nodes in his/her neck

↓

Are they fixed and non-tender or painful and mobile?

Fixed, non-tender → Look for enlarged lymph nodes elsewhere and assess spleen and liver size clinically and radiographically → Blood count and blood film → Lymphocytosis: measure immunoglobulins and flow cytometry for B-cell 'clonal' lymphocytosis → Diagnosis: chronic lymphocytic leukaemia

Small, painful, mobile nodes → Look for infection on head and neck and infection or tumour in mouth/throat

OUTCOME

Because of increasing nodes, decreasing energy and night sweats, the patient was treated with a combination of chemotherapy and antibodies to CLL cells and had an excellent response. He did not require immunoglobulin replacement therapy, but was vaccinated. He was advised to have 'cold sores' treated promptly and to contact his doctor immediately if he was in contact with an individual with chicken pox or shingles. He remained at work and was able to resume his 18 holes of golf weekly. He wore the same shirt and bow tie to the annual golf dinner without any difficulty.

Suggested reading

Rozman, C. & Montserrat, C. (1995) Chronic lymphocytic leukemia. *New England Journal of Medicine*, **333** (16), 1052–7.

Mauro, F.R., Foa, R., Cerretti, R. *et al.* (2000) Autoimmune haemolytic anemia in chronic lymphocytic leukaemia: clinical, therapeutic and prognostic features. *Blood*, **95** (9), 2786–92.

Cheson, B.D. (ed.) (2001) *Chronic Lymphoid Leukemias*. Marcel Dekker, Inc., New York, USA.

Matutes, E., Morilla, R. & Catovsky, D. (2001) Immunophenotyping. In: *Practical Haematology* (eds S.M. Lewis, B.J. Bain & I. Bates), 9th edn, pp. 297–314. Churchill Livingstone, London, UK.

Schiller, G.J. (ed.) (2003) *Chronic Leukemias and Lymphomas: Biology, Pathophysiology and Clinical Management*. Humana Press, New Jersey, USA.

A man with fatigue and a sore throat

Bernard, a 40-year-old plumber, noticed a decrease in energy for a few weeks and has had a sore throat for almost a week. He normally works 11 hours a day and often does emergency calls at weekends. He also goes hill walking at weekends, but has not been able to do this for 3 weeks. He went to his family doctor because he had a sore throat, noticed a rash on his legs and he was bleeding from his gums for a few days, which frightened him.

Q1 What could cause these symptoms and signs?

A The loss of energy and the pallor could be due to anaemia. The petechial rash suggests an inflammation of the small blood vessels (vasculitis) or a reduced platelet count. The sore throat, which was 'erythematous', suggests an infection.

The combination of these signs and symptoms suggests a bone marrow problem resulting in failure of the normal blood functions, i.e. anaemia, bleeding and infection.

Q2 What should be done next?

A A physical examination.

He appeared healthy but looked pale and had a petechial rash (purpura) on his legs (Fig. 12.1). His throat was red and inflamed looking. There was no lymphadenopathy and his spleen and liver were not enlarged.

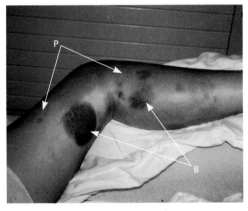

Figure 12.1 Ecchymoses (bruising) (B) and petechiae (P).

Q3 What is the meaning of 'purpura'?

A 'Purpura' means bleeding into the skin. If it causes small pinpoint red spots they are known as 'petechiae' and if the bleeding becomes confluent it is called an 'ecchymosis'. To distinguish this from a dilated blood vessel gentle pressure is applied to the area. If bleeding has occurred into the skin (purpura) the lesion will not change colour. If the lesion is due to a dilated blood vessel it will 'blanch' (lose its colour) and the red colour will return in a few seconds when the pressure is removed.

Q4 What investigations should be done?

A A full blood count (Table 12.1), blood film (Fig. 12.2) and biochemical screen (Table 12.2).

> **Key point**
> He should be asked to wait for the results because of the probability of a serious underlying pathology.

Table 12.1 Full blood count

	Patient's results	Normal range
Hb	9.0 g/dl	13.5–18.0 g/dl
MCV	87.0 fl	83.0–99.0 fl (μm^3)
WBC	35.4×10^9/l	$4.0–11.0 \times 10^9$/l (10^3/μl)
Neutrophils	1.0×10^9/l	$2.0–7.5 \times 10^9$/l (10^3/μl)
Lymphocytes	34.4×10^9/l	$1.5–3.5 \times 10^9$/l (10^3/μl)
Platelets	20.0×10^9/l	$150–450 \times 10^9$/l (10^3/μl)

Table 12.2 Biochemical screen

	Patient's results	Normal range
Creatinine	125 µmol/l	50–115 µmol/l (0.5–1.7 mg/dl)
Urate	600 µmol/l	150–470 µmol/l (3.0–8.0 mg/dl)
Lactic dehydrogenase (LDH)	1000 IU/l	230–450 IU/l

The laboratory technician said that many of the 'lymphocytes' looked like leukaemic 'blasts' but she wanted the haematologist to review the blood film. The platelet count was low. She suspected the patient had acute leukaemia (Fig. 12.2).

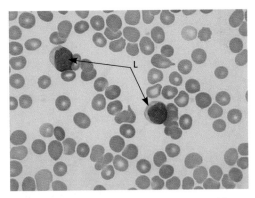

Figure 12.2 A blood film showing leukaemia blasts (L) with no evidence of maturation.

Q5 **What disease could explain the symptoms, signs and blood findings?**

A Acute leukaemia may cause dramatic symptoms and signs within a few days or weeks.

Q6 **What happens in acute leukaemia to produce these symptoms, signs and blood findings?**

A Normally, the bone marrow (the factory which produces the blood cells) produces red blood cells, white cells and platelets in a very orderly fashion so that the numbers of these cells in the blood remains relatively constant throughout life (Table 12.3).

Table 12.3 Lifespan of blood cells

Type of cell	Lifespan
Red cell	120 days
Neutrophil	4–6 hours
Lymphocyte	Years
Platelet	7–10 days

> **Key point**
> If the factory fails to produce normal blood cells the rate of reduction in the cell numbers in the blood will reflect the 'normal' lifespan of that cell. Clinically, this means a reduction in the number of neutrophils first and then the platelets and red cells.

A Leukaemic cells fail to differentiate (Figs 12.3 and 12.4), that is, they fail to develop the normal function expected of them. They also have a reduced rate of apoptosis.

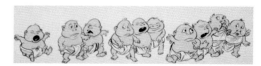

Figure 12.4 Simulated acute leukaemia, where there is failure of maturation and function.

The major mechanisms for failure of maturation and reduced rate of apoptosis are acquired genetic abnormalities that include gene translocations, deletions and mutations. These genetic aberrations influence intracellular signalling, cell growth, differentiation and apoptotic rates. Leukaemia cells are called 'blasts'.

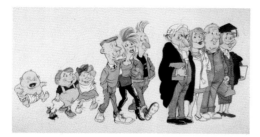

Figure 12.3 Normal maturation and function.

A Leukaemia cells 'inhibit' the development of normal cell differentiation in the non-involved cells in the bone marrow, probably by releasing cytokines.

A Tell the patient that he has a serious blood disease and arrange immediate admission to hospital.

The patient was admitted to a specialist haematology unit. The history was verified. There was no known exposure to marrow toxins or drugs that could cause these blood findings. The physical findings were confirmed and the optic fundi were examined for haemorrhage. His gums appeared hypertrophic (increase in gum tissue around the base of the teeth) (Fig. 12.5). His blood pressure was checked.

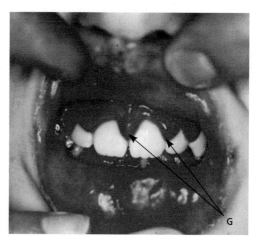

Figure 12.5 Gum hypertrophy (G).

A A low platelet count can cause bleeding into the 'macula', which can cause blindness. Fresh bleeding in the fundi may predict bleeding into the brain and therefore needs immediate management. His blood pressure was 125/75 mmHg (120/80 mmHg).

> **Key point**
> An elevated blood pressure together with a low platelet count increases the risk of bleeding.

Q11 What is the relevance of the gum hypertrophy?

A In some forms of leukaemia the leukaemic cells invade the gum tissue and cause it to swell. This is usually found in leukaemias of 'monocytic' origin. Other tissues can also be invaded (Fig. 12.6).

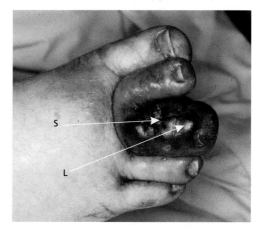

Figure 12.6 Leukaemic infiltration into the toe (L); the suture marks (S) are from the biopsy site.

Q12 What drugs should be specifically enquired about?

A The patient should be specifically asked about ingestion of aspirin or anti-inflammatory drugs within the preceding week. These drugs are in very common usage and people often forget that they have taken them.

> **Key point**
> Aspirin does not influence the platelet count but may cause bleeding because of inhibition of platelet function. Aspirin, and to a lesser extent non-steroidal anti-inflammatory drugs, inhibit the cyclooxygenase pathway and interfere with platelet function. This reaction is not reversible and therefore platelet function will not recover until new platelets are released from the bone marrow.

A A bone marrow sample should be taken from the posterior iliac crest and sent to the laboratory for all of the investigations. The blood count should be repeated, as should the liver, bone and renal biochemical profiles (Table 12.2).

A A high cell turnover will result in an elevated LDH and urate and cause renal impairment, leading to a high creatinine level.

The patient was given intravenous fluids to reduce the urate and creatinine levels and the nurses were instructed not to give any intramuscular injections (a low platelet count could cause severe bleeding). Allopurinol (a xanthine oxidase inhibitor) was given to reduce the urate level. A sample of urine was sent for microbiological analysis and a chest radiograph was carried out. He was instructed in mouth care to minimize the risk of further infection. He was given broad-spectrum antibiotics because he was febrile (temperature 38.5°C). The urine did not contain any granulocytes and the chest radiograph was normal.

A Because patients with low granulocyte counts cannot mount the normal inflammatory response the usual signs of infection are commonly absent. Treatment with antibiotics should be given 'empirically' for a presumed infection.

He was given a platelet transfusion and the site of the bone marrow aspiration was carefully monitored for bleeding.

The bone marrow examination confirmed a diagnosis of acute myeloid leukaemia (Fig. 12.7).

> ### Key point
> The diagnosis of bacterial infection depends, to a large extent, on the signs of inflammation. Swelling, redness and pain are the common signs of infection because of the infecting organism and the granulocyte and monocyte response. Granulocytes in the urine or an 'infiltrate' (shadow) on a chest radiograph are signs of infection in a normal individual.

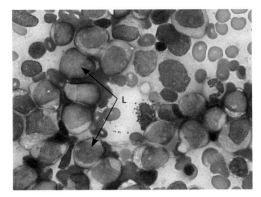

Figure 12.7 A bone marrow aspirate, showing replacement of normal marrow with leukaemia blasts (L).

A The type of leukaemia is important because it will influence the treatment and probable outcome.

Leukaemias are typed by trying to determine how the leukaemic cell would have developed under normal circumstances. Because the leukaemic cells are 'undifferentiated' the morphology is not always conclusive in making a diagnosis of the type of leukaemia and a number of other investigations must be carried out.

A Table 12.4 shows the methods used to classify leukaemia.

Table 12.4 Classifying leukaemia

Method	Observation
Morphology	The appearance of the leukaemia cells on a glass slide (see Fig. 12.2).
Cytochemistry	Special stains to try to identify primitive cell constituents, which might provide a clue as to the possible differentiation pathway that had been blocked in that cell.
Flow cytometry	A study of the surface antigens on the leukaemic cell.
Cytogenetics	Determination of the aberrant genetic material (chromosomes) in the leukaemia cell (Fig. 12.8).
Molecular genetics	Study of the DNA of the leukaemic cell. This is also useful to 'track' the patient after therapy to see if the leukaemia has been eradicated (Fig. 12.9).

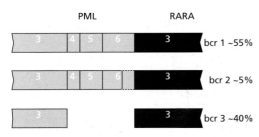

Figure 12.8 An illustration of translocations between chromosomes 15 and 17 in acute promyelocytic leukaemia.

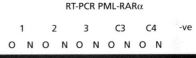

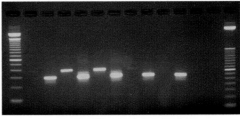

O = outer (1st round PCR),

N = nested (2nd round PCR), C3 = control −3 dilution,

C4 = control −4 dilution; -ve = negative control

Figure 12.9 A gel following RT-PCR showing in lanes 1, 2 and 3 the abnormal 15:17 translocation in acute promyelocytic leukaemia. Lanes 1, 2 and 3 contain patient material. Lanes C3 and C4 are controls.

The significance of the diagnosis was explained to the patient and his wife and he was given combination chemotherapy.

A The frequency is the same in adults as in children. Most adults with leukaemia are over the age of 50 years at the time of diagnosis.

The common cell of origin in adult leukaemia is 'myeloid' (derived from granulocyte or monocyte precursor cells) and in children is 'lymphoid'.

Key point

Acute lymphoblastic leukaemia (ALL) was one of the first malignancies to be cured by combination chemotherapy including corticosteroids. The treatment was developed in the late 1960s and 1970s and the current experience indicates a cure rate of approximately 80%. Because of a propensity for ALL cells to invade the CSF and brain, prophylaxis is given early in the treatment of the leukaemia with intrathecal chemotherapy or irradiation. Patients who relapse may benefit from stem cell transplantation.

Q19 Can you now construct an algorithm for a man with fatigue and sore throat?

A Yes.

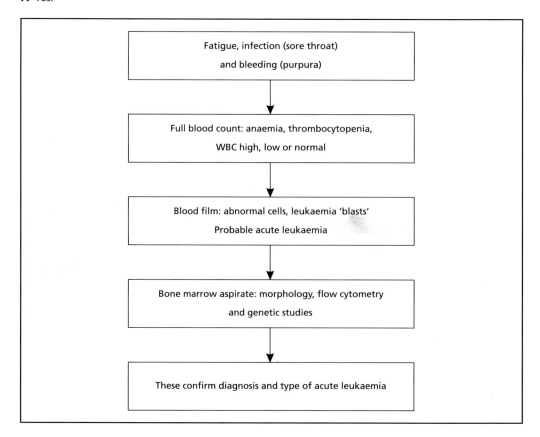

Fatigue, infection (sore throat) and bleeding (purpura)

↓

Full blood count: anaemia, thrombocytopenia, WBC high, low or normal

↓

Blood film: abnormal cells, leukaemia 'blasts' Probable acute leukaemia

↓

Bone marrow aspirate: morphology, flow cytometry and genetic studies

↓

These confirm diagnosis and type of acute leukaemia

OUTCOME

The patient was treated with combination chemotherapy, which achieved a complete remission. He subsequently received two further courses of combination chemotherapy and returned to work 6 months after the original diagnosis.

Suggested reading

Pui, C.H. (1995) Childhood leukemias. *New England Journal of Medicine*, **332** (24), 1618–30.

Löwenberg, B. & Burnett, A.K. (1999) Acute myeloid leukaemia in adults. In: *Textbook of Malignant Haematology* (eds L. Degos, D. Linch & B. Löwenberg), pp. 743–69. Martin Dunitz, London, UK.

Löwenberg, B., Downing, J.R. & Burnett, A. (1999) Acute myeloid leukemia. *New England Journal of Medicine*, **341** (14), 1051–62.

Hoffbrand, A.V., Pettit, J.E. & Moss, P.A.H. (2001) *Essential Haematology*, 4th edn. Blackwell Science, Oxford. See Chapter 12: Acute leukaemias.

Henderson, E., Lister, T.A. & Greaves, M.F. (2002) *Leukaemia*, 7th edn. Saunders, Philadelphia, USA.

A farmer with a broken rib

A 58-year-old farmer called Tom stumbled and fell while herding his sheep. He complained of severe rib pain. His wife put him to bed and gave him aspirin. He had difficulty sleeping because of the pain, so the next day they attended the family doctor's surgery.

The family doctor had known Tom for many years. As well as the pain in his ribs, his wife told the doctor that her husband had been complaining of low back pain for about 6 months. The patient volunteered that he felt very tired at the end of the day and often 'nodded off' to sleep in a chair after his evening meal.

The doctor remarked that he thought Tom 'looked a little smaller' than when he had seen him a few months earlier. He also thought Tom looked a little pale.

Q1 What might explain his symptoms?

A Fatigue is difficult to evaluate and in this age group it could be due to heart failure, anaemia or cancer. Arthritis would explain his back pain but is unlikely to make him pale. He may have an underlying neoplasm. The loss of height may suggest osteoporosis and collapse of a vertebral body. The combination of back pain and pallor should make a bone marrow problem a consideration.

The family doctor recommended radiographs of his back and ribs. Since the farmer was very busy he delayed going for the radiographs. A few weeks later he began to complain of nausea and shortness of breath. He developed a cough, which caused severe rib pain.

Q2 How does this information help to interpret his symptoms?

A He has broken ribs with a secondary chest infection because the pain makes it difficult for him to take a deep breath.

The family doctor was quite worried and referred him to the local accident and emergency department.

A Take a history about previous illness, especially chest infections, smoking habit, alcohol consumption and medications.

He had been very well until this episode. He had two chest infections in the last 6 months, which required treatment with antibiotics, which was unusual for him. He had smoked 20 cigarettes a day for all his adult life and had a glass of whiskey before retiring to bed. He drank 4–5 pints of beer at weekends. He denied coughing blood and had not experienced hoarseness or any change in his voice. This information was verified by his wife.

Q4 What diagnoses could be considered?

A Lung cancer is a definite possibility. His smoking history and recent chest infections are suspicious findings. Back pain could be due to metastases from lung cancer. Lung cancer could also explain his pallor, as it may be associated with anaemia. Multiple myeloma can cause bone pain and anaemia.

On examination his pulse was 120/min. His blood pressure was 120/60 mmHg and he had a fever of 38°C. He was pale and dehydrated. He had a marked kyphosis and there was decreased air entry with coarse crackles at the left lung base.

Q5 What investigations should be ordered?

A A full blood count (Table 13.1), blood film (Fig. 13.1), and renal, liver and bone profiles (Table 13.2).

Table 13.1 Full blood count

	Patient's results	Normal range
Hb	8.5 g/dl	13.5–18.0 g/dl
MCV	90.0 fl	83.0–99.0 fl (μm^3)
White cell count	11.6×10^9/l	4.0–11.0×10^9/l (10^3/μl)
Platelet count	160×10^9/l	140–450×10^9/l (10^3/μl)
Differential white cell count	Normal	

Table 13.2 Biochemical results

	Patient's results	Normal range
Serum creatinine	215.0 mmol/l	50–115 μmol/l (0.5–1.7 mg/dl)
Calcium	3.36 mmol/l	2.20–2.70 mmol/l (8.6–10.3 mg/dl)
Albumin	26.0 g/l	35–50 g/l (3.5–5.0 g/dl)
Total protein	95.5 g/l	60–80 g/l (6.0–8.0 g/dl)

The blood film (Fig. 13.1) showed 'rouleaux' formation.

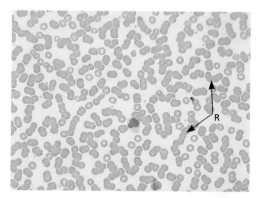

Figure 13.1 Blood film showing 'rouleaux' formation (R).

Q6   What do these abnormalities suggest?

A Tom is anaemic and the 'rouleaux' formation of the red cells reflects an elevation of plasma fibrinogen or immunoglobulins.

> **Key point**
> 'Rouleaux' formation means that the red cells appear like coins stacked upon each other. This happens because the red cells are covered with fibrinogen or immunoglobulin which inhibit the charge which usually makes red cells repel each other.

Q7   What are the major abnormalities in the biochemistry profile?

A The blood levels of calcium and creatinine are elevated. The total protein level is elevated and the albumin level is decreased.

The elevated creatinine suggests renal failure, which could be caused by the hypercalcaemia. The increased total protein and the low albumin suggest a disturbance of liver function.

The chest radiograph shows that he has a left-sided pneumonia. In addition, he has a fractured rib (Fig. 13.2) and a multiple 'lytic' lesion in the humerus (Fig. 13.3). His lumbar spine shows evidence of osteoporosis (decrease in mineralization) and collapse of a number of vertebrae.

The vertebral collapse has led to the kyphosis.

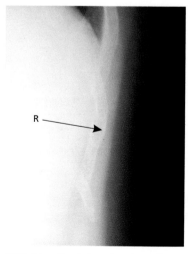

Figure 13.2 A localized view showing a fractured rib (R).

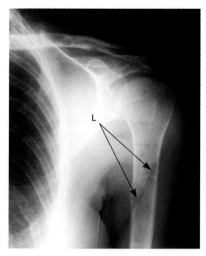

Figure 13.3 A radiograph showing multiple lytic lesions in the humerus (L).

Q8 When would a radionuclide bone scan be preferable?

A Radionuclide scans are very informative when osteoblastic lesions are being investigated. Osteolytic lesions are best detected by plain radiography or MRI.

Q9 Which tumours frequently give rise to bone lesions?

A Bone metastasis occurs from cancer of the prostate, breast, lung, kidney, bladder and thyroid. Metastatic tumours to bone are much more common than primary bone tumours. Multiple myeloma causes osteolytic lesions of bone.

Q10 What cancer could the patient have, which would be causing all his problems?

A Metastatic cancer could be causing his problems. However, some of the clinical and laboratory parameters make an alternative diagnosis more likely.

Q11 Which parameters may be useful in pointing to the likely diagnosis?

A The combination of bone pain, infection, anaemia, renal failure (raised plasma creatinine) and the raised total protein make the diagnosis of multiple myeloma (cancer of plasma cells) seem likely.

A Measurement of serum immunoglobulins (Table 13.3).

Table 13.3 Immunoglobulin levels

Serum immunoglobulins	Patient's results	Normal range (male)
IgG	66.0 g/l (6600 mg/dl)	6.40–15.22 g/l (700–1450 mg/dl)
IgA	0.20 g/l (20 mg/dl)	0.48–3.44 g/l (70–370 mg/dl)
IgM	0.15 g/l (15 mg/dl)	0.29–1.86 g/l (30–210 mg/dl)

Q13 **What cells normally produce immunoglobulins and what does the term 'monoclonal band' mean?**

A B-lymphocytes normally produce immunoglobulins (antibodies), which bind foreign antigens, e.g. bacteria and viruses. Immunoglobulins represent the output of millions of different plasma cells. The normal response consists of molecules of immunoglobulins with different mixtures of κ and λ light chains. A monoclonal (M) band reflects the synthesis of immunoglobulin from a single clone of plasma cells and, therefore, one light chain type. These monoclonal proteins are called 'paraproteins'.

Q14 **What do these results suggest?**

A A raised IgG level and reduced IgA and IgM levels suggest a disease affecting B cells.

A Electrophoresis of the serum proteins (Figs 13.4 and 13.5).

> **Key point**
> In multiple myeloma the monoclonal band is most commonly IgG (60%).

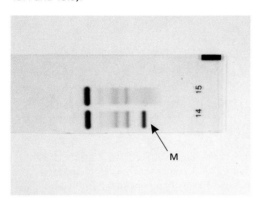

Figure 13.4 A scan of the serum proteins. Proteins are placed on a supporting matrix and separated according to size and charge. The dense staining in the immunoglobulin region suggests that there is a 'monoclonal' protein present (M).

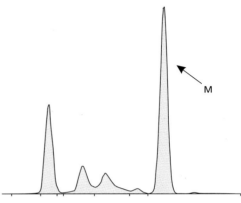

Figure 13.5 A densitometry scan of the serum proteins; M shows the monoclonal band.

Q16 What other test should be done to prove monoclonality?

A Immunofixation of the serum.

Antibodies to IgG, IgA, IgM, κ and λ are used to show the protein has a single light chain.

Q17 What is the significance of the low IgA and IgM?

A Most cancer cells are non-functional. In multiple myeloma the abnormal B cells produce a 'monoclonal', non-functional protein and also fail to produce a normal antibody response. Therefore, the patient has hypogammaglobulinaemia (a low level of immunoglobulins). This explains the low IgA and IgM. The low levels of immunoglobulins cause increased susceptibility to infection, which is the presenting feature in approximately 25% of patients with multiple myeloma.

> **Key point**
> Patients with hypogammaglobulinaemia are most prone to infections with encapsulated bacterial organisms. These patients have very poor antibody responses, especially to polysaccharide antigens such as those in the bacterial cell walls. The absence of antibodies directed against the bacterial capsule limits the ability of phagocytic cells to ingest and kill the bacteria. The most common infections in people with hypogammaglobulinaemia are due to *Streptococcus pneumoniae* or *Haemophilus influenzae*.

A Bone marrow aspirate (Fig. 13.6), and β2-microglobulin levels.

The combination of blood, marrow, biochemical and immunological findings confirms a diagnosis of multiple myeloma.

> **Key point**
> Serum β2-microglobulin (β2-M) was raised at 3.0 mg/l (normal: 1.05–2.05 mg/l). This is the single most powerful predictor of survival in patients with multiple myeloma.

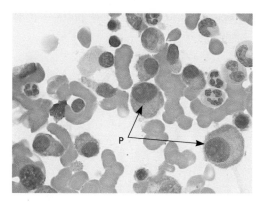

Figure 13.6 A bone marrow aspirate, showing multiple malignant plasma cells (P) with dark blue cytoplasm and an eccentric nucleus. The blue staining cytoplasm indicates immunoglobulin synthesis.

A β2-M is the light chain of the class 1 histocompatibility antigen and is expressed on the surface of all nucleated cells. The increase in β2-M in multiple myeloma is a reflection of the tumour mass. It is excreted by the kidneys and is also elevated in renal failure.

Renal failure occurs in about 25% of patients with multiple myeloma.

A A monoclonal gammopathy of uncertain significance (MGUS). Patients with MGUS usually have a relatively low paraprotein level. They have a normal Hb and renal function. 10% of the population over the age of 70 have an MGUS. No treatment is indicated for MGUS but follow-up is necessary, as approximately 25% of patients with MGUS will ultimately develop multiple myeloma.

A Yes.

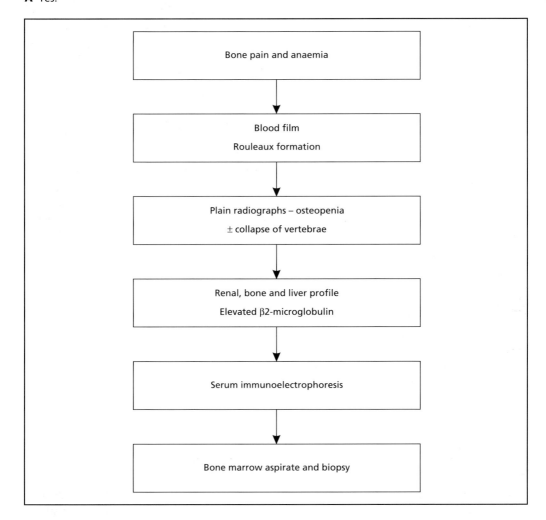

OUTCOME

Tom was admitted to hospital. He was given intravenous fluids to relieve his dehydration, hypercalcaemia and renal failure. In addition, he was treated with a combination of corticosteroids and a bisphosphonate for the hypercalcaemia. He also received intravenous antibiotics for his chest infection and analgesia for his bone pain. Over the next few days his condition markedly improved with normalization of his creatinine and calcium. He was given six courses of combination chemotherapy followed by an autogolous stem cell graft.

One year later he is feeling very well and doing a full day's work on the farm. He no longer has any bone pain. His most recent immunoglobulins show that his paraprotein is no longer detectable.

On his last clinic visit he was delighted to tell you that 'Daisy the cow' won first prize at his local agricultural show.

Suggested reading

Bataille, R. & Harousseau, J.L. (1997) Multiple myeloma. *New England Journal of Medicine*, **336** (23), 1657–64.

Malpas, J.S., Bergsagel, D.E., Kyle, R.A. *et al.* (eds) (2004) *Myeloma: Biology and Management*, 3rd edn. Oxford University Press, Oxford.

Kyle, R.A., Morie, M.D., Gertz, A. *et al.* (2003) Review of 1027 patients with newly diagnosed multiple myeloma. *Mayo Clinical Proceedings*, **78**, 21–33.

Trpos, E., Politu, M. & Rahemtulla, A. (2003) New insights into the pathophysiology and management of bone disease in multiple myeloma. *British Journal of Haematology*, **123**, 758–69.

(2003) Multiple myeloma and other plasma cell neoplasms www.cancer.gov/cancerinfo/pdq/treatment/myeloma/healthprofessional, National Cancer Institute.

A medical student who complained of bone pain following alcohol ingestion

Ann, an 18-year-old medical student, presented to the haematology clinic with a 4-week history of fatigue and general malaise. She had been to her family doctor on two occasions during this period for a sore throat, for which she received antibiotics. She had noticed a swelling on the right side of her neck about 3 weeks ago.

Q1 What could be causing these symptoms?

A Recurrent sore throat in a young person with fever and swelling in the neck suggests a viral infection. However, the degree of fatigue and malaise should make you suspicious of a more serious underlying disease such as a lymphoma.

Q2 What viral infection would you suspect?

A Infectious mononucleosis.

Infectious mononucleosis, also called glandular fever, is an acute infection commonly seen in adolescence and in young adults. The manifestations are fever, sore throat, and enlarged lymph glands and the cause is the Epstein–Barr virus (EBV). It is usually self-limiting and is spread commonly by intimate oral contact, such as kissing (it is sometimes referred to as the 'kissing' disease).

Q3 What should be done next?

A A full history should be taken, with emphasis on weight loss, anorexia, fever or night sweats. Any change in size of the swelling, pain or tenderness should be enquired about.

She admitted to a weight loss of 4 kg and night sweats on six occasions during the last month. The swelling had increased in size but was never painful and was not tender to touch. She had an unproductive cough for 4 days. She has mild asthma, for which she takes bronchodilators with good effect. She noticed bone pain on a few occasions after consuming alcohol. There was no other history apart from the usual childhood illnesses.

Q4 What is the significance of the night sweats, weight loss and bone pain induced by alcohol?

A They are highly suggestive of Hodgkin's disease. Although fever, sore throat and malaise can be found in a viral infection, such as infectious mononucleosis, bone pain induced by alcohol, although rare, is a finding which appears to be specific to patients with Hodgkin's disease.

Q5 What should be done next?

A A full physical examination.

On examination she was pale and appeared unwell. She had a mass in the right supraclavicular area, which measured 2 × 2 cm, was non-tender and fixed. There were no other enlarged lymph nodes and the liver and spleen were normal. She had a temperature of 38°C.

Q6 What do the physical findings suggest?

A The pallor suggests anaemia and the fixed non-tender mass suggests a malignancy.

Q7 What type of anaemia would be most common in a girl of this age?

A Iron-deficiency anaemia.

Q8 What questions should be asked if iron deficiency is suspected?

A A full dietary history, details of menstrual blood loss and any other evidence of bleeding.

A low iron intake is common in adolescence and can contribute to iron deficiency. Bleeding, particularly menorrhagia, is also a common cause of iron deficiency in this age group.

Q9 What is the significance of the fever?

A A viral infection or an upper respiratory tract bacterial infection could cause a fever (she has a history of asthma and complained of an unproductive cough); however, fever can be a manifestation of lymphoproliferative diseases.

Q10 What investigations should be done?

A A full blood count (Table 14.1), a blood film, biochemical screen (see Table 14.2), erythrocyte sedimentation rate (ESR), viral screen, a chest radiograph, and analysis of the sputum for evidence of infection.

The ESR was 60 mm/hour (normal, female: 0–15 mm/hour).

The blood film showed an increased number of platelets but no other abnormalities.

Table 14.1 Full blood count

	Patient's results	Normal values (female)
Hb	8.3 g/dl	11.5–16.4 g/dl
MCV	69 fl	83–99 fl (μm^3)
WBC	$8.1 \times 10^9/l$	$4–11 \times 10^9/l$ ($10^3/\mu l$)
Neutrophils	$5.4 \times 10^9/l$	$2.0–7.5 \times 10^9/l$ ($10^3/\mu l$)
Lymphocytes	$2.7 \times 10^9/l$	$1.5–3.5 \times 10^9/l$ ($10^3/\mu l$)
Platelets	$746 \times 10^9/l$	$140–450 \times 10^9/l$ ($10^3/\mu l$)
Reticulocytes	$85 \times 10^9/l$	$50–100 \times 10^9/l$ (0.5–15%)

Q11 What blood film abnormalities would you expect to see in infectious mononucleosis?

A The presence of atypical mononuclear cells.

Q12 What could be the cause of the high platelet count?

A An increased platelet count is commonly found as a response to acute haemorrhage. It can also be found in malignancies and may be a manifestation of myeloproliferative diseases, e.g. chronic myeloid leukaemia (see Case 10), polycythaemia rubra vera (see Case 16) or iron deficiency (see Case 1).

Q13 What is the significance of the elevated ESR?

A The elevation is a non-specific finding in infections or malignancies.

The ESR measures the rate of sedimentation of red cells in a tube. Red cells are normally kept apart by van der Waal's forces. In patients with infection or malignancies, high levels of immunoglobulin (antibodies) or fibrinogen (a plasma coagulation protein) may inhibit these forces, allowing the red cells to stick together.

A Serum protein electrophoresis and a coagulation screen.

The serum protein electrophoresis shows a polyclonal gammopathy. This indicates a normal response to infection, but can be a non-specific finding in malignancy. The coagulation screen revealed a fibrinogen of 12 g/l (normal: 1.5–4.0 g/l), which explains the raised ESR. The synthesis of fibrinogen may be increased in malignancies.

The viral screen, including EBV serology, was negative, so excluding a diagnosis of infectious mononucleosis.

The chest radiograph (Fig. 14.1) showed enlargement of the right paratracheal nodes.

Table 14.2 Biochemical results

	Patient's results	Normal values
Bilirubin	5 µmol/l	0–17 µmol/l (0.3–1.1 mg/dl)
Alk phos	376 IU/l	40–120 IU/l
GGT	100 IU/l	5–40 IU/l
LDH (lactic dehydrogenase)	240 IU/l	230–450 IU/l
Ferritin	150 µg/l	20–300 µg/l (20–300 ng/ml)

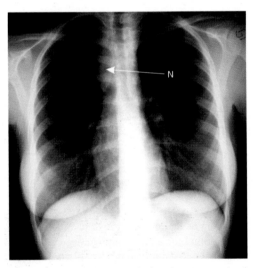

Figure 14.1 Chest radiograph showing paratracheal lymphadenopathy (N).

A She is anaemic with a low MCV, suggesting iron deficiency or the anaemia of chronic disease. The normal serum ferritin excludes iron deficiency. The high platelet count could be associated with a malignancy as there is no clinical evidence of acute haemorrhage. Her liver blood tests are abnormal, suggesting a viral infection or malignancy. The chest radiograph confirms enlarged lymph nodes in the neck and upper mediastinum. These results together with her symptoms suggest Hodgkin's disease.

> **Key point**
> Fever, night sweats and weight loss are known as B symptoms and are commonly found in Hodgkin's disease, non-Hodgkin's lymphoma and chronic lymphocytic leukaemia.

A She should be admitted to hospital immediately.

A Bone marrow aspirate and biopsy (Fig. 14.2) and a CT scan of thorax and abdomen (Fig. 14.3).

The bone marrow aspirate and biopsy showed increased iron stores in keeping with the diagnosis anaemia of chronic disease. The CT of thorax and abdomen showed adenopathy in the anterior mediastinum (Fig. 14.3).

> **Key point**
> Bone marrow involvement in Hodgkin's disease (Fig. 14.2) is extremely uncommon and occurs in less than 5% of patients.

The anaemia of chronic disease is characterized by a low MCV but normal ferritin and bone marrow iron stores. It is commonly seen in association with malignancy or chronic infectious diseases such as tuberculosis. There is a block in the transport of iron into the developing red cell precursors, giving rise to red cells which are deficient in iron in a patient who has adequate iron stores.

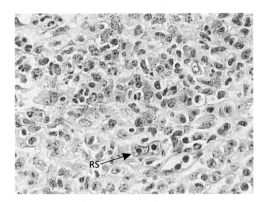

Figure 14.2 Bone marrow with Reed–Sternberg cells (RS) (i.e. Hodgkin's disease).

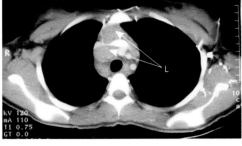

Figure 14.3 CT scan of thorax showing lymphadenopathy in the superior mediastinum (L).

Q18 What should be done next?

A A lymph node biopsy.

A lymph node biopsy revealed nodular sclerosing Hodgkin's disease (Fig. 14.4).

Hodgkin's disease is a malignancy most
commonly of B cell origin. It is manifested by
enlarged lymph nodes, hepatosplenomegaly
and B symptoms. The classic cell associated with
Hodgkin's disease is the Reed–Sternberg cell.
There is evidence of EBV infection in many patients with Hodgkin's disease, but a direct causa-
tive role has not been demonstrated.

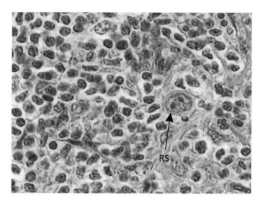

Figure 14.4 Lymph node biopsy shows Reed–
Sternberg cells (RS) and collagen bands: nodular
sclerosing Hodgkin's disease.

> **Key point**
> Hodgkin's disease is most frequently seen in
> adolescents and young adults, but there is a
> second peak after the age of 50 years.

Q19 How do the investigations influence the management?

A The extent of the disease will influence the
type of management.

Q20 What are the principles of management of Hodgkin's disease?

A Hodgkin's disease is one of the earliest malignancies to be cured by combination chemotherapy. However, extensive nodal disease may
also require radiotherapy.

> **Key point**
> The long-term cure rate for Hodgkin's disease
> is now so good that the emphasis is now being
> placed on limiting the toxicity of the therapy.

A Yes.

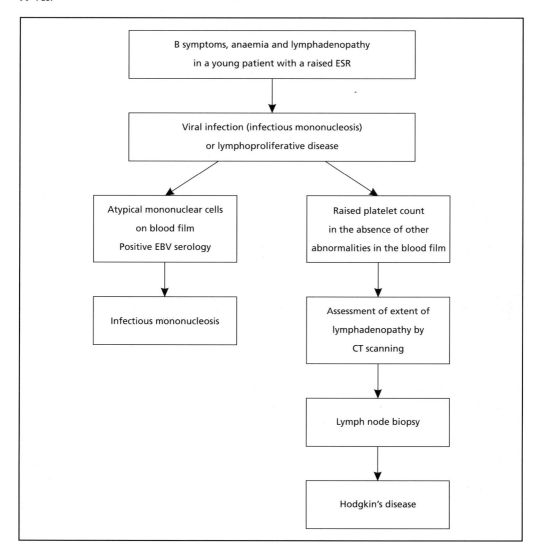

OUTCOME

She was treated with combination chemotherapy, to which she had a complete response. She returned to her medical studies 6 months from the time of her diagnosis. She is currently in her third medical year and remains in complete remission from her disease.

Suggested reading

Hasenclever, D. & Diehl, V. (1998) A prognostic score for advanced Hodgkin disease. *New England Journal of Medicine*, **339**, 1506–1514.

Kadin, M.E. (2000) Pathology and histogenesis of Hodgkin disease. In: *Hematology. Basic Principles and Practice* (eds R. Hoffman, E.J. Benz, Jr, S.J. Shattil, B. Furie, H.J. Cohen, L.E. Silberstein & P. McGlave), 3rd edn, pp. 1229–41. Churchill Livingstone, New York, USA.

Portlock, S.C., Glick, J. & Kadin, M.E. (2000) Hodgkin disease: Clinical manifestations, staging, and therapy. In: *Hematology. Basic Principles and Practice* (eds R. Hoffman, E.J. Benz, Jr, S.J. Shattil, B. Furie, H.J. Cohen, L.E. Silberstein & P. McGlave), 3rd edn, pp. 1241–62. Churchill Livingstone, New York, USA.

Berthe, M.P., Aleman, M.D., Raemaekers, J.M.M. *et al.* (2003) Involved-field radiotherapy for advanced Hodgkin lymphoma. *New England Journal of Medicine*, **348** (24), 2396–406.

Diehl, V., Franklin, J., Pfreundschuh, M. *et al.* (2003) Standard and increased-dose BEACOPP chemotherapy compared with COPP-ABVD for advanced Hodgkin disease. *New England Journal of Medicine*, **348** (24), 2386–95.

A woman with discomfort under her left arm

Mary is a 53-year-old Caucasian woman who works as a part-time secretary. Over the last 3 weeks she has felt a discomfort under her left arm (axilla) when washing herself. In addition to her work, she regularly babysits for her two small grandchildren. She now finds it more tiring. Fifteen years earlier she suffered from breast cancer in her right breast. She says that it was a small tumour and that she was treated with radical mastectomy (surgical removal of her breast and associated lymph nodes) and radiotherapy. She has been well since. She used to smoke but had stopped when the breast cancer was discovered and drinks only an occasional glass of wine.

Q1 What could be the cause of her clinical symptoms and signs?

A The discomfort (Mary has never used the word pain) is presumably associated with the local feeling of 'enlargement'. This could be due to a cyst, enlarged lymph nodes due to a malignancy of the lymphoid system or metastases from a cancer, possibly a recurrence of her original disease.

Q2 What should you concentrate on when taking the history?

A A better definition of the symptoms and clinical signs, as well as the duration. Ask specific questions and link them to events in her personal life or a well-known public event. Had the swelling ever been painful and was it increasing in size? Was the swelling tender? Did she notice weight loss, fever or night sweats?

The swelling was not painful but probably had increased in size recently. Her weight was stable and there was no history of night sweats.

Q3 What should be done next?

A A full physical examination.

She appeared healthy and the only abnormal physical finding was a nodal mass in the left axilla.

A A full blood count (Table 15.1), blood film (Fig. 15.1), biochemical screen and viral screen, a chest radiograph, a mammogram (radiological examination of the breast to detect cancers which cannot be felt clinically) and an ultrasound examination of the left axilla and of the abdomen.

The blood film showed an increased number of 'atypical' cleaved lymphocytes.

Table 15.1 Blood count

	Patient's results	Normal range (female)
Hb	13.9 g/dl	11.5–16.4 g/dl
WBC	8.9×10^9/l	$4.0–11.0 \times 10^9$/l (10^3/µl)
Lymphocytes	6.0×10^9/l	$1.5–3.5 \times 10^9$/l (10^3/µl)
Neutrophils	2.9×10^9/l	$2.0–7.5 \times 10^9$/l (10^3/µl)
Platelets	210×10^9/l	$140–450 \times 10^9$/l (10^3/µl)

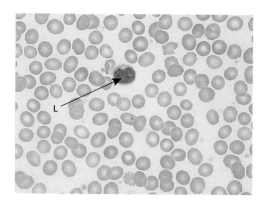

Figure 15.1 'Atypical' lymphocytes (L).

A It is possible that it is a recurrence of her breast cancer (this is, understandably, her primary worry); however, the lymphocytosis suggests a blood disorder, therefore a lymph node biopsy is indicated. There is no immediate danger, but further investigation is needed. She should continue with her normal daily activities. She should be reviewed as soon as the results of the tests become available.

Epstein–Barr (EBV) serology was negative and the biochemical screening showed a moderate increase in LDH to 605 IU/l (normal: 230–450 IU/l), with the other values being normal.

The mammography, chest radiograph and ultrasound of the abdomen were negative. The ultrasound examination of the left axilla confirmed the enlarged lymph node.

What do you think is going on?

A The possibility of breast cancer recurrence has been ruled out and the most frequent viral infections have been excluded. There is further confirmation of abnormal lymph node enlargement in the left axilla, with a concomitant increase in LDH. A slight increase in lymphocytes was also noted, although the remaining haematological values were all normal.

Q7 **What diagnosis can be suspected?**

A Having excluded other possibilities (breast cancer recurrence, viral infections), an enlarged axillary lymph node, coupled to an increase in LDH strongly suggests the presence of an underlying lymphoma. Only a biopsy can provide a precise diagnosis.

> **Key point**
> Lactic dehydrogenase, LDH, is a ubiquitous enzyme found in all nucleated cells. It is found in the blood when cells die. This can be as a result of cancer, infarction of any tissue, premature destruction of red blood cells (haemolysis) or ineffective erythropoiesis (vitamin B_{12} or folate deficiency). It is a prominent finding in non-Hodgkin's lymphoma and the degree of elevation of the LDH is indicative of the 'aggressiveness' of the lymphoma.

Q8 **Why does the patient have a slight increase in lymphocytes (lymphocytosis), with other haematological values within the normal range?**

A If the diagnosis of a lymphoma is confirmed, the slight lymphocytosis could be due to the presence of lymphoma cells in the blood. This requires further investigation.

Q9 **How should the patient be managed?**

A Arrange to see the patient and her husband to explain that she needs to undergo an excision lymph node biopsy as soon as possible in order to make a diagnosis. This can be done as an outpatient under local anaesthesia. She should continue with her various activities and the biopsy will be arranged with the surgeon within the following week.

The procedure takes place 4 days later and the biopsy is sent unfixed to the pathologist. The conclusions of the histological examination are that the patient suffers from a non-Hodgkin's lymphoma of follicular origin (Fig. 15.2).

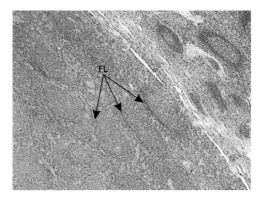

Figure 15.2 A lymph node with a follicular lymphoma (FL).

What should the patient be told?

A The lymph node biopsy has confirmed that she has non-Hodgkin's lymphoma (NHL). I would explain that this is a malignancy of the lymphoid tissues that most often affects lymph nodes, that there are different forms of non-Hodgkin's lymphoma and that she does not have any of the more aggressive forms. Her disease can be treated successfully and that she should be referred to a haematologist as soon as possible.

Q11 **What do you think the haematologist would do?**

A The physical findings were confirmed and nothing further emerged from the personal and family history.

The pathological evaluation of the lymph node confirmed that the patient suffered from a follicular non-Hodgkin's lymphoma (NHL). The pathological cells were of B-cell origin and were 'clonal' as they showed an Igκ light chain restriction.

Non-Hodgkin's lymphomas are a group of diseases which provide us with an insight into the mechanisms of malignancy.

Lymph nodes are removed (excision biopsy means removing the complete node, instead of a piece of the node) for pathological examination and the cells made into a suspension and analysed by flow cytometry. The node may also be cut into thin sections and immunological investigations carried out to demonstrate the 'clonality' of the malignant cells.

Lymphomas are derived from B or T cells (the majority are derived from B cells). To demonstrate 'clonality', i.e. that the malignant cells are derived from a single cell, a functional test has been developed. B cells normally produce immunoglobulins (Ig). In a reactive or inflammatory (non-malignant) node, B cells produce Igs of different light chain types. In a malignant node the Ig will be of a single light chain type, κ or λ (light chain restriction), indicating its origin from a single cell.

Another finding of great importance is that commonly there is transfer of genetic material from one chromosome to another in the malignant cells. Chromosomal material from chromosome 14 is 'translocated' to chromosome 18, resulting in a resistance to apoptosis (programmed cell death) in the malignant cells. This gives us a clue to the mechanisms involved in the malignant cell and opens up new possibilities for treatment. These translocations and 'clonality' in lymphoma cells can be demonstrated by flow cytometry, immunocytochemistry and genetic analysis.

Q12 **Based on the diagnosis made, how could the increased number of lymphocytes in the patient's blood be more precisely investigated?**

A Flow cytometry. Since the neoplastic cells are B cells with an Igκ chain restriction, these cells can be easily looked for in the blood through a simple flow cytometry evaluation.

It was found that the patient had lymphoma cells in her blood.

A A CT scan of the abdomen and thorax and a bone marrow biopsy will help to evaluate the extent of disease.

The CT scan of the thorax was negative, while the CT of the abdomen showed enlarged lymph nodes (Fig. 15.3).

The bone marrow biopsy showed a small infiltration of Igκ lymphoma cells.

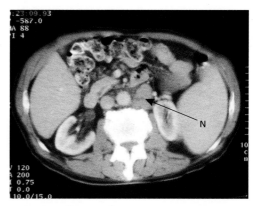

Figure 15.3 CT scan of the thorax was negative, while the CT of the abdomen showed enlarged retroperitoneal and para-aortic lymph nodes (N).

Q14 What are the practical implications of all these investigations?

A To subdivide NHL into 'indolent' (slow growing) or 'aggressive' (rapidly growing) forms, as these bear important prognostic implications. Follicular lymphoma patients most often fall within the indolent subtype and, less frequently, under the aggressive subtype.

Key point

Although the incidence is increasing, we do not know the aetiology of most lymphomas. However, a number of lymphomas occur where a viral aetiology has been demonstrated. Dr Denis Burkitt was the first to demonstrate the viral cause of a particular lymphoma in Africa. This was a lymphoma found in the jaw of children and was subsequently shown to be caused by the Epstein–Barr virus (EBV). EBV, however, is not a cause of the common B or T cell lymphomas found in adults. The EBV virus has been implicated in the lymphomas found in HIV infected patients.

A The choice of treatment depends on the stage of the disease and the age and general health of the patient. Radiotherapy alone can be utilized for patients in the initial stages of the disease. Chemotherapy is usually utilized for patients with more advanced disease.

More recently, the combination of chemotherapy and the monoclonal antibody Rituximab (induces apoptosis in malignant B cells via the CD20 antigen) has been successfully utilized. In younger patients 'autografting' can also be considered.

Q16 Can you now construct an algorithm for the investigation of a patient with a large lymph node?

A Yes.

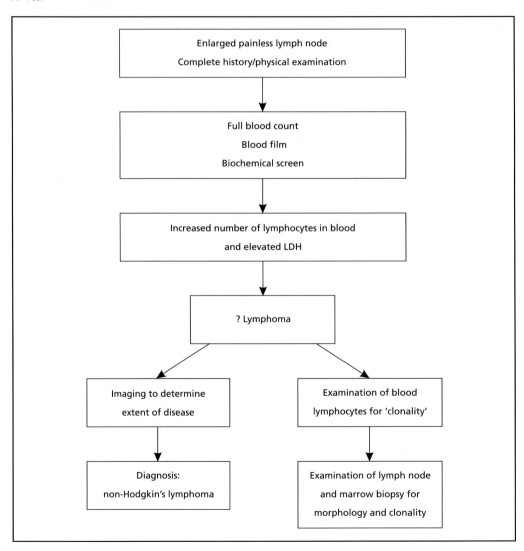

OUTCOME

The patient was treated with a combination of chemotherapy, after which she had a complete disappearance of symptoms and clinical and laboratory signs. However, monitoring of her disease indicated persistence of malignant B cells in her bone marrow after completing the chemotherapy programme. She was then given the anti-CD20 antibody, which induced a complete remission of her disease. Mary returned to 100% fitness, to work and enjoyed looking after her grandchildren again.

Suggested reading

Reiser M. & Diehl, V. (2002) Current treatment of follicular non-Hodgkin's lymphoma. *European Journal of Cancer*, **38** (9), 1167–1172.

Kipps, T.J. (2002) Advances in classification and therapy of indolent B-cell malignancies. *Seminars in Oncology*, **29** (1 Suppl. 2), 98–104.

Rambaldi, A., Lazzari, M., Manzoni, C. *et al.* (2002) Monitoring of minimal residual disease after CHOP and rituximab in previously untreated patients with follicular lymphoma. *Blood*, **99** (3), 856–62.

Schiller, G.J. (ed.) (2003) *Chronic Leukemias and Lymphomas, Biology, Pathophysiology and Clinical Management*. Humana Press, New Jersey, USA.

Staudt, L.M. (2003) Molecular diagnosis of the hematologic cancers. *New England Journal of Medicine*, **348**, 1777–85.

A red-faced man with a 'smoker's cough'

A 65-year-old male was encouraged to go to his family doctor by his wife because she thought his cough was getting worse and he seemed a little confused lately. He retired 1 year ago from a clerical job in an insurance company. For the last 6 months he felt a little 'muzziness' and that the crossword, which he had completed every day for the last 30 years, was now becoming difficult. Some days he did not bother even reading the newspaper! He had been a cigarette smoker all his adult life and he thought his chronic cough, worse in winter, had deteriorated recently.

Q1   What might cause these symptoms?

A Chronic bronchitis and/or emphysema, since he had smoked cigarettes for all of his adult life and has a chronic cough.

Q2   What would a change in the pattern of a 'smoker's cough' make you think of?

A A change in the pattern of a 'smoker's cough', hoarseness or coughing blood (haemoptysis) are highly suspicious of lung cancer.

Q3   How could a diagnosis of lung cancer be linked with the other symptoms?

A Lung cancer can spread (metastasize) to the brain and produce symptoms of poor concentration or 'muzziness'.

A Take a full history with particular reference to hoarseness, haemoptysis, weight loss and precisely what the patient's wife meant by a change in the pattern of his cough. Ask about a history of high blood pressure or respiratory tract infections and a family history of cancer.

The patient had about one respiratory tract infection yearly requiring antibiotics. He denied any change in his voice, haemoptysis, weight loss or a real change in the pattern of his cough. His cough did not keep him awake at night and he was trying to stop smoking.

He had two children, a son aged 40 and a daughter aged 42, both of whom were alive and well.

A A complete physical examination, focusing on the cranial nerves and central nervous system. Measure the blood pressure; examine the urine and optic fundi.

There was no papilloedema (presence indicates raised intracranial pressure which could indicate a primary brain tumour or metastasis). He looked plethoric (Fig. 16.1). The blood pressure was elevated at 160/100 mmHg. The cranial nerves and central nervous system were intact. A few crackles were audible in both lung bases. The only other abnormality was an enlarged spleen, palpable 4 cm below the left costal margin in quiet inspiration (Figs 16.2 and 16.3). There was no blood or protein in the urine.

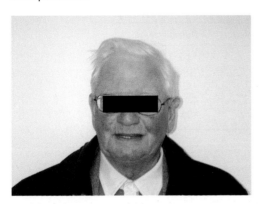

Figure 16.1 A plethoric face.

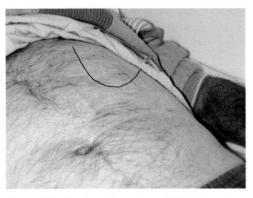

Figure 16.2 The tip of the spleen visible below the left coastal margin.

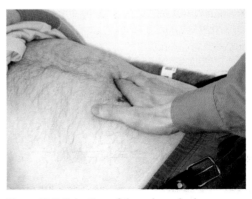

Figure 16.3 Palpation of the enlarged spleen.

What else might you ask in view of his physical appearance?

A Ask the patient and his wife if they had noticed a change in the patient's physical appearance in the last year, in particular if his face was more 'purple-red' than it used to be.

Ask the patient if he has a photograph of himself taken a few years ago.

Q7 **What investigations should be done?**

A A chest radiograph and ultrasound examination of the abdomen. A full blood count (Table 16.1), blood film and a biochemical screen.

> **Key point**
>
> He should stop smoking immediately (nicotine substitutes or other supportive measures are frequently required). If a patient stops smoking at 65 years and lives for another 10 years he/she will significantly reduce the risk of developing lung cancer.

Table 16.1 Full blood count

	Patient's results	Normal range
Hb	19.5 g/dl	13.5–17.5 g/dl
MCV	70.0 fl	76–96 fl (μm^3)
RBC	7.0×10^{12}/l	$4.5–6.5 \times 10^{12}$/l ($10^6/\mu l$)
WBC	13.5×10^9/l	$4.0–11.0 \times 10^9$/l ($10^3/\mu l$)
Platelets	625×10^9/l	$150–450 \times 10^9$/l ($10^3/\mu l$)

Q8 **How should the patient be managed?**

A He should return in a few days for a further blood pressure measurement and the results of the blood tests.

The radiograph showed some hyperinflation of the chest, a normal heart size and no evidence of lung cancer. The ultrasound examination con-firmed an enlarged spleen. His blood pressure remained elevated at 150/100 mmHg.

Occasional large platelets were noted on the blood film. There was an elevated uric acid level of 520 μmol/l (normal: 150–470 μmol/l or 3.0–8.0 mg/dl).

A The haemoglobin and red cell count are both increased, so the patient has erythrocytosis. The platelet count is also elevated, so there could be a bone marrow problem causing an excess production of red cells and platelets. The patient also has a large spleen, suggesting that there is some fundamental disturbance of the haematological system. The elevated uric acid could have been present for a long time and may reflect idiopathic hyperuricaemia or increased cell turnover.

A Lung cancer could cause his cough and his 'muzziness' because of metastases in his brain. It is unusual to have a large spleen with metastatic cancer. The erythrocytosis could be secondary to chronic lung disease and hypoxia as a result of his cigarette smoking.

Some lung cancers secrete a hormone with 'erythropoietin-like' activity causing the raised red cell count. A raised platelet count can occur with any malignancy.

Other possibilities include diseases which cause a reduction in blood oxygen levels (hypoxaemia) such as a right to left shunt in the heart, heavy cigar smoking, chronic obstructive airways disease, a congenital high-affinity haemoglobin, or a renal cyst producing 'erythropoietin-like' hormones. Polycythemia rubra vera, a disease where there is overproduction of red cells (and sometimes white cells and platelets), in the bone marrow should also be considered.

> **Key point**
> Red cell production is a precisely regulated phenomenon (Fig. 16.4).

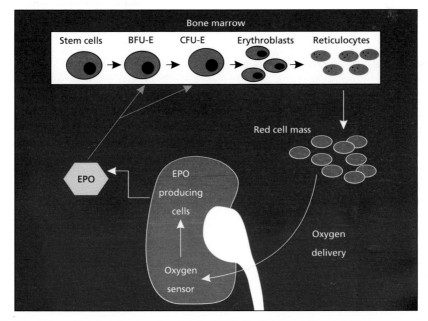

Figure 16.4 The interactions between erythropoietin (EPO), the kidney and oxygenation.

A He should be referred to hospital immediately for further investigations.

The patient was given an appointment for the following week to see a haematologist.

Q12   What would the haematologist do?

A Repeat the history and physical examination, which confirmed the plethoric appearance, enlarged spleen and elevated blood pressure.

Q13   What investigations were carried out?

A Sputum was examined for malignant cells, which, if present, would indicate lung cancer.

The chest radiograph findings were confirmed. Pulse oximetry (Fig. 16.5) was carried out.

This revealed an oxygen saturation of 97% (normal: 96–100%).

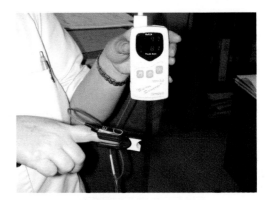

Figure 16.5 Pulse oximetry.

Q14   How reliable is pulse oximetry in detecting hypoxaemia in the patient?

A Very reliable. Thus, hypoxaemia is not the reason for the increased red cell count. Arterial blood gases should be measured if the oximetry is abnormal and the patient investigated to elucidate the cause.

> **Key point**
> The commonest cause of hypoxaemia is chronic obstructive airways disease secondary to chronic cigarette smoking.

A Measure the level of erythropoietin (EPO) in the plasma and the blood and plasma volume (Table 16.2).

The principle of blood and plasma volume measurement is that of dilutional analysis. A small amount of radiolabelled substance, usually radioactive chromium, is added to a small volume of the patient's red blood cells, and then re-injected. The blood volume can be calculated from the dilution in the whole blood of the patient. Plasma volume can be similarly measured using radiolabelled albumin.

Table 16.2 EPO levels and blood and plasma volume

	Patient's results	Normal range
Red cell mass	50.1 ml/kg	20–30 ml/kg
Plasma volume	43.7 ml/kg	40–50 ml/kg
Total blood volume	93.8 ml/kg	60–80 ml/kg
Erythropoietin (EPO)	8.5 IU/ml	6.0–25.0 IU/ml

Q16 How can these results be interpreted?

A The EPO level is normal. The red blood cell mass is increased and the plasma volume is normal, confirming that there is an excess production of red cells.

Q17 How useful is the measurement of EPO in making a diagnosis?

A It is sometimes useful. If there is a hypoxaemic state the levels of EPO are elevated, reflecting the increased drive to produce red cells. However, if a tumour or a renal cyst is secreting EPO, the serum levels are not elevated and samples from the blood vessel draining the tumour or directly from the renal cyst are taken. In polycythemia rubra vera the serum levels of EPO are usually normal or decreased.

Q18 What do the results so far indicate?

A The patient has an overactive bone marrow as a reason for erythrocytosis other than hypoxia.

Q19 What other investigations would the haematologist perform at this stage?

A A bone marrow biopsy (Fig. 16.6).

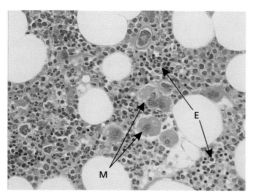

Figure 16.6 A bone marrow biopsy, showing erythroid hyperplasia (E) and increased numbers of megakaryocytes (M).

The bone marrow findings support a diagnosis of polycythemia rubra vera (PRV).

PRV is a disease usually seen in people over the age of 60 years. It is due to a clonal expansion in the marrow, leading to excess production of red blood cells, granulocytes and platelets. ('Clonal' means derived from a single clone of bone marrow stem cells.) Like other clonal disorders of the marrow, there may be chromosomal abnormalities. Deletions (partial loss) of chromosome 20 are the commonest findings.

Q20 What clinical problems would he experience if untreated?

A Vascular problems in the arterial and venous circulation. The increased number of circulating red cells and red cell mass will increase the blood viscosity. The increased platelet numbers, cigarette smoking and high blood pressure will also increase the risk of arterial vascular problems.

Q21 What other investigation could support the diagnosis?

A Measurement of red cell colony growth from marrow 'stem cells'.

Normally, or in patients with erythrocytosis due to hypoxia, red cell colonies will grow only in the presence of EPO. In PRV, red cell colonies will grow without the addition of EPO, i.e. spontaneous growth.

Q22 Can you now construct an algorithm to investigate a patient with erythrocytosis?

A Yes.

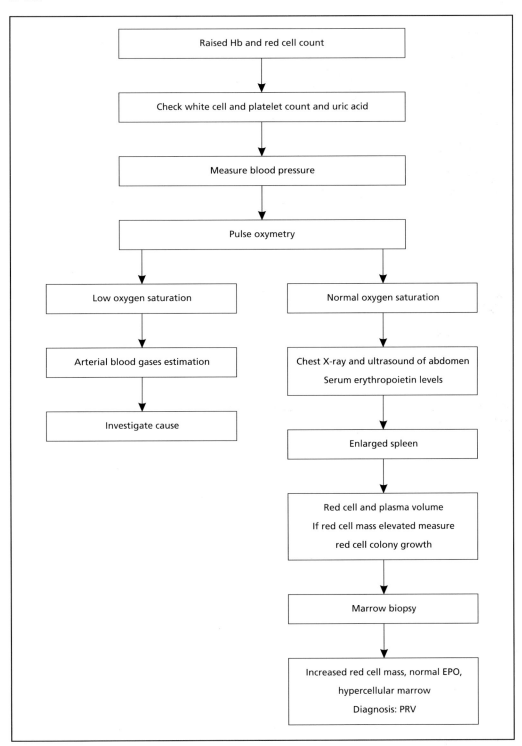

OUTCOME

A diagnosis of PRV was made. His blood pressure was treated and he was given oral chemotherapy with hydroxyurea until his platelet count returned to normal (150–450 × 10^9/l or 10^3/µl). He was venesected at weekly intervals until his haemoglobin returned to normal (13.5–17.5 g/dl) and encouraged to stop smoking. His symptoms disappeared and he returned to his daily crossword puzzles.

> **Key point**
>
> Avoid the use of diuretics when treating high blood pressure in patients with PRV as they will decrease the plasma volume, therefore increasing the haematocrit and increasing the risk of vascular events. Remember: do not venesect a patient if the platelet count is elevated.
>
> The platelet count will rise further following the venesection and could cause a 'stroke'.

Suggested reading

Gruppo Italiano Studio Policitemia (1995) Polycythemia vera: the natural history of 1213 patients followed for 20 years. *Annals of Internal Medicine*, **123**, 656–64.

Means, R.T., Jr (1999) Polycythemia vera. In: *Wintrobe's Clinical Hematology* (eds G.R. Lee, J. Foerster, J. Lukens, F. Paraskevas, J.P. Greer & G.M. Rodgers), 10th edn, Vol. 2, pp. 2374–89. Williams and Wilkins, Baltimore, USA.

Hoffbrand, A.V., Pettit, J.E. & Moss, P.A.H. (2001) *Essential Haematology*, 4th edn. Blackwell Science, Oxford. See Chapter 17: Myeloproliferative disorders.

Lewis, S.M. (2001) Diagnostic radionuclides in haematology. In: *Practical Haematology* (eds S.M. Lewis, B.J. Bain & I. Bates), 9th edn, pp. 315–37. Churchill Livingstone, London, UK.

Tefferi, A. (2003) Polycythemia vera: a comprehensive review and clinical recommendations. *Mayo Clinical Proceedings*, **78**, 174–94.

A young lady who had suddenly started bruising

Mary, a 28-year-old web-site designer, went to her doctor because she had noticed bruising on her arms and legs for 3–4 days. The bruises were not painful and were increasing in number every day.

A Spontaneous bruising could be due to a decreased platelet count (thrombocytopenia), abnormal platelet function or inflammation of blood vessels resulting in leakage of red cells into the skin (vasculitis).

A A full history, with particular emphasis on recent (viral) infection and medications. She had no fever or other evidence of infection and was taking no medications.

A A physical examination.

The examination revealed a healthy looking young woman with bruising and petechiae on her arms and legs (Fig. 17.1). There was no other abnormality; specifically, the spleen was not palpable.

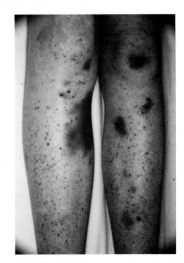

Figure 17.1 Extensive bruising and petechiae.

A A full blood count (Table 17.1), blood film (Fig. 17.2), coagulation and biochemical screen.

The patient was requested to return later that afternoon for the results.

Table 17.1 Full blood count

	Patient's result	Normal range
Hb	12.0 g/dl	11.5–16.4 g/dl
WBC	5×10^9/l	$4.0–11.0 \times 10^9$/l (10^3/μl)
Neutrophils	3.5×10^9/l	$2.0–7.5 \times 10^9$/l (10^3/μl)
Lymphocytes	1.5×10^9/l	$1.5–3.5 \times 10^9$/l (10^3/μl)
Platelets	15×10^9/l	$140–450 \times 10^9$/l (10^3/μl)

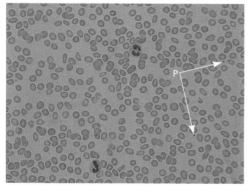

Figure 17.2 A blood film showing reduced platelets (P). In a normal individual, 10–25 platelets are expected in a field of this magnification.

The coagulation screen was normal and the blood film confirmed a reduced platelet count (Fig. 17.2).

Q5 How can the full blood count and coagulation screen be interpreted?

A The platelet count is obviously extremely low. This would probably explain why the girl has had spontaneous bruising. The Hb and white cell count are normal, making bone marrow failure an unlikely diagnosis. The coagulation screen is not influenced by the platelet count as a platelet substitute is added to the test material. Therefore, thrombocytopenia does not cause a prolonged prothrombin time (PT) or activated partial thromboplastin time (APTT).

Q6 What should be done next?

A The patient should be referred to a specialist immediately.

A The patient should be advised not to take aspirin or any anti-inflammatory drugs.

She should be advised to rest that evening and see the specialist the following day.

The next day she was seen by a haematologist.

> **Key point**
>
> Aspirin or any anti-inflammatory drugs inhibit platelet function due to inhibition of cyclooxygenase. The inhibition induced by aspirin is irreversible and platelet function will only recover following synthesis and release of new platelets from the bone marrow.

Q8 What would the haematologist do?

A Repeat the blood count and examine the blood film (Fig. 17.2). Repeat the physical examination.

> **Key point**
>
> Remember to include examination of the retina as part of the physical examination. Bleeding into the retina can cause blindness if it occurs in the area of the macula, but also can be a 'window' to look at small blood vessels and predict the possibility of an intracranial bleed.

The blood counts were unchanged (Table 17.1) and the blood film (Fig. 17.2) confirmed a low platelet count. There were no abnormal white cells present, making the diagnosis of leukaemia unlikely.

Q9 What further tests would the haematologist carry out?

A A biochemical screen and an ultrasound of the abdomen.

The biochemical screen was normal and the abdominal ultrasound revealed a normal spleen size with no intra-abdominal masses or lymphadenopathy.

Q10 What other serological investigation should be carried out?

A A screening test for HIV infection.

Q11 What precautions should be taken before carrying out this test?

A The patient should be informed of the possible diagnosis in the case of the test being positive. A full history of possible exposure to HIV and patient consent should be obtained.

Q12 How would you manage this patient?

A The patient should be admitted to hospital and orders given that she should not receive any intramuscular injections (Fig. 17.3), aspirin or non-steroidal anti-inflammatory drugs.

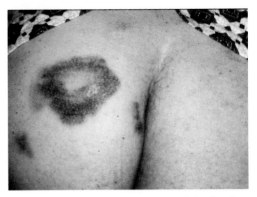

Figure 17.3 A large haematoma at an injection site in a patient with a low platelet count.

Q13 What would the haematologist do next?

A Carry out a bone marrow aspirate and biopsy (Fig. 17.4).

The bone marrow aspirate and biopsy revealed an increased number of platelet precursors (megakaryocytes) and no abnormal cells.

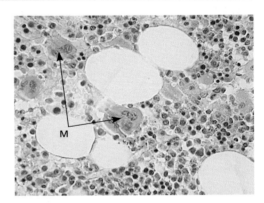

Figure 17.4 Bone marrow, showing increased numbers of megakaryocytes (M).

Q14 How can you connect the appearance of the bone marrow with the low platelet count and the absence of a large spleen?

A The increased numbers of megakaryocytes (platelet precursors) in the bone marrow suggest that platelet production is normal. The decreased number of platelets in the blood, therefore, suggests that there is premature destruction of platelets. Platelet numbers may be decreased in the presence of a large spleen, as pooling may occur.

A Immune thrombocytopenic purpura (ITP).

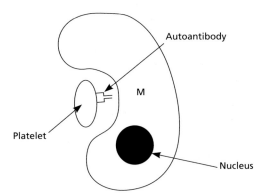

Figure 17.5 A macrophage (M) in the spleen engulfing an autoantibody and the platelet to which it is attached.

In ITP an autoantibody is formed, for reasons unknown, against a protein on the platelet membrane. The antibody adheres to the platelet membrane and is phagocytosed by macrophages in the reticuloendothelial system, primarily in the spleen. When engulfing the Fc receptor of the autoantibody, the macrophage also engulfs the platelet and the platelet is, therefore, destroyed (Fig. 17.5). If the rate of destruction of platelets exceeds the compensatory increased production by the bone marrow (the marrow can increase the production by 6–7 times) the platelet count will fall and levels may go to $<10 \times 10^9/l$ ($10^3/\mu l$).

Q16 **What drugs in common use can be associated with a low platelet count?**

A Quinine, the antibiotics trimethoprim–sulpha-methoxazole (Septrin) and rifampicin.

Q17 **What drug commonly used in hospitals can cause a low platelet count?**

A Heparin.

Heparin-induced thrombocytopenia–thrombosis syndrome (HITTS) may occur if patients are given heparin to prevent or treat venous throm-

bosis. The syndrome occurs because heparin induces platelet clumping leading to further thrombosis, both venous and arterial, and a low platelet count.

Q18 **At what platelet level is there a danger of spontaneous intracranial bleeding?**

A It depends on the mechanism of the low platelet count.

If the low platelet count is due to premature destruction, the young platelets, which are released from the bone marrow, have excellent function

and bleeding rarely occurs into the brain even if the platelet count is $<10 \times 10^9/l$ ($10^3/\mu l$).

If the low platelet count is due to bone marrow failure, then a platelet count of $<10 \times 10^9/l$ ($10^3/\mu l$) may result in a high risk of intracranial bleeding.

A In a patient with ITP the spleen is not enlarged. Although there is increased activity in the spleen, the organ is always of normal size.

> **Key point**
> The finding of an enlarged spleen in a patient with a low platelet count indicates a diagnosis other than ITP.

Q20 What syndrome may present with thrombocytopenia and an enlarged spleen?

A Systemic lupus erythematosus (SLE).

In this autoimmune disease, which is seen predominantly in young females, skin rashes, arthralgia and renal impairment are seen. The low platelet count is immune mediated.

Q21 What diagnostic test result would exclude a diagnosis of SLE?

A Absence of anti-DNA antibodies.

The clinical course of ITP differs in children and adults (Table 17.2).

Table 17.2 ITP in children and adults

Children	Adults
ITP in children is usually of acute onset, commonly follows a viral infection and is nearly always self-limiting. Treatment is rarely required.	In adults, ITP is nearly always chronic (a duration of >14 days), is rarely preceded by a viral infection and rarely recovers without treatment.

Q22 What are the principles of management of ITP?

A In children, observation and conservative management is usually adequate. In adults, if a low platelet count is accompanied by bleeding, then treatment should be initiated in hospital using corticosteroids or intravenous immunoglobulins.

Q23 What are the potential hazards of giving immunoglobulin derived from human donor plasma?

A There is always a risk of transmission of known or unknown viruses, other infectious agents, e.g. prions, when products derived from human plasma are used. The combination of intensive screening, including a detailed medical history, and measures taken for the inactivation of viruses reduces the risk substantially (see Case 20).

Q24 In the event of failure of medical therapy and persistent thrombocytopenia and bleeding, what further interventions might be considered?

A Splenectomy (Fig. 17.6).

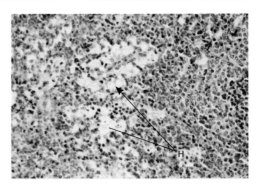

Figure 17.6 A histological section of a spleen removed from a patient with ITP, showing an increase in histiocytes which are engulfing platelets H.

Q25 How does removal of the spleen compromise the patient?

A Individuals without a spleen are more liable to overwhelming infection with Gram-positive en- capsulated bacteria (*Streptococcus pneumonia* and *Haemophilus influenzae*).

Q26 What precautions should be taken prior to removal of the spleen?

A Vaccination against the above.

Q27 What other precaution should be taken after the spleen is removed?

A Administration of penicillin or erythromycin.

Q28 For how long should this treatment be administered after splenectomy?

A For life.

A Yes.

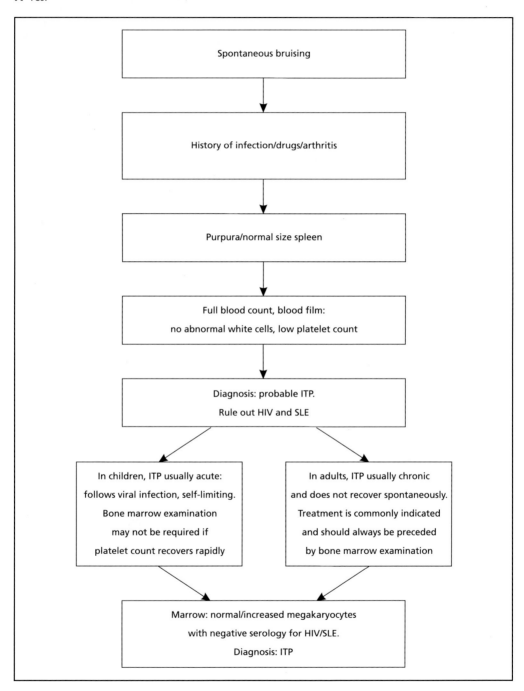

Spontaneous bruising

↓

History of infection/drugs/arthritis

↓

Purpura/normal size spleen

↓

Full blood count, blood film:
no abnormal white cells, low platelet count

↓

Diagnosis: probable ITP.
Rule out HIV and SLE

In children, ITP usually acute:
follows viral infection, self-limiting.
Bone marrow examination
may not be required if
platelet count recovers rapidly

In adults, ITP usually chronic
and does not recover spontaneously.
Treatment is commonly indicated
and should always be preceded
by bone marrow examination

Marrow: normal/increased megakaryocytes
with negative serology for HIV/SLE.
Diagnosis: ITP

OUTCOME

Because of the bleeding, she was treated with corticosteroids and immunoglobulin. Severe thrombocytopenic bleeding persisted, so a splenectomy was carried out after vaccination. Penicillin was prescribed post-operatively. She remains well with a normal platelet count 2 years later.

> **Key point**
> The diagnosis of ITP is one of exclusion as there is no specific test for this condition.

Suggested reading

George, J.N., Woolf, S.H., Raskob, G.E. *et al.* (1996) Idiopathic thrombocytopenic purpura: a practice guideline developed by explicit methods for the American Society of Hematology. *Blood*, **88**, 3–40.

Hoffbrand, A.V., Pettit, J.E. & Moss, P.A.H. (2001) *Essential Haematology*, 4th edn. Blackwell Science, Oxford. See Chapter 19: Bleeding disorders caused by vascular and platelet abnormalities.

George, J.N., Raskob, G.E., Shar, S.R. *et al.* (2001) Drug-induced thrombocytopenia: a systematic review of published case reports. *Annals of Internal Medicine*, **129**, 886–90.

British Committee for Standards in Haematology, General Haematology Task Force (2003) Guidelines for the investigation and management of idiopathic thrombocytopenic purpura in adults, children and in pregnancy. *British Journal of Haematology*, **120**, 574–96.

Delivery of a baby boy that went wrong

Anne was admitted to the delivery suite in her local Maternity Hospital. Because she failed to 'progress in labour' forceps were used to deliver the head of the baby. After delivery the midwife noticed that the baby had a large haematoma (blood under the skin) on the scalp.

Q1 What should the midwife do?

A Call the neonatologist immediately.

Q2 What should the neonatologist do?

A A full physical examination of the baby.

Physical examination was normal apart from the haematoma on the scalp (Fig. 18.1).

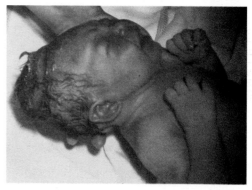

Figure 18.1 Haematoma on the scalp. Reproduced with kind permission from E.P. Mauser-Bunschoften.

Q3 What should the neonatologist do next?

A Take a history from the mother.

Q4 What questions should be asked to find out if the patient has a history of abnormal bleeding?

A Did she ever have bleeding following dental extraction or surgery? Did bleeding occur into joints or was easy bruising a feature?

She said that as far as she was aware there was no family history of abnormal bleeding.

> **Key point**
> Coagulation factor deficiencies typically have abnormal bleeding into muscles and joints. Bleeding due to a platelet deficiency causes bleeding from mucosal surfaces and bruising. Excessive menstrual blood loss may be the only evidence of a bleeding disorder.

Q5 How helpful is a patient's history when trying to assess menorrhagia (excessive menstrual blood loss)?

A Frequently, it is unhelpful. Each woman's definition of menorrhagia can be different.

> **Key point**
> Menorrhagia is defined as greater than 80 ml blood loss on three consecutive periods; laboratory-based assays are the only way to measure it accurately.

Q6 What should be done next?

A Interview the father of the baby, asking if there is a family history of abnormal bleeding in his family.

Many young mothers are unmarried and are not in regular contact with the child's father. Anne was not aware of any history of abnormal bleeding in him or his family.

Q7 Why is the family history of the mother or father important?

A Because the bleeding occurred at the time of delivery it is possible that the child has a congenital bleeding disorder. As congenital bleeding disorders are commonly familial, a family history would be useful to confirm this possibility.

A A full blood count and platelet count (Table 18.1) and coagulation screen (Table 18.2).

Table 18.1 Blood count

	Baby's results	Normal range (0–1 month)
Hb	11.6 g/dl	13.4–19.9 g/dl
MCV	120 fl	88–123 fl (µm^3)
Platelets	440 × 10^9/l	140–450 × 10^9/l (10^3/µl)

Table 18.2 Coagulation screen

	Patient's results	Normal range
Prothrombin time, PT	14.2 sec	12–15 sec
Activated partial thromboplastin time, APTT	82.0 sec	26–35 sec
Thrombin time, TT	14.8 sec	14–16 sec
Fibrinogen	2.90 g/l	1.67–3.99 g/l (150–360 mg/dl)

Q9 How can the full blood count be interpreted?

A The baby is anaemic and the red cells are larger than normal. This may reflect bleeding, which has occurred into the baby's scalp. The platelet count is normal, excluding thrombocytopenia as a cause of the bleeding.

Q10 What further tests could be done to elucidate the cause of the baby's anaemia?

A A reticulocyte count (Table 18.3).

Table 18.3 Reticulocyte count

	Patient's result	Normal range
Reticulocytes	134 × 10^9/l	20–100 × 10^9/l (0.2–1.5%)

Q11 How can this result be interpreted?

A The reticulocyte count is increased as a response to the bleeding and causes the high MCV, as reticulocytes are larger than normal red cells.

A The APTT is prolonged and the PT is normal. This indicates an abnormality of the 'intrinsic clotting system', which is measured by the APTT (Fig. 18.2). This is probably due to haemophilia, as a deficiency of factor VIII or IX would result in a prolonged APTT with a normal PT and also cause bleeding.

> **Key point**
>
> The PT and APTT are not influenced by the platelet count, as a substitute for platelets is added during the testing of a patient's plasma.

INTRINSIC PATHWAY

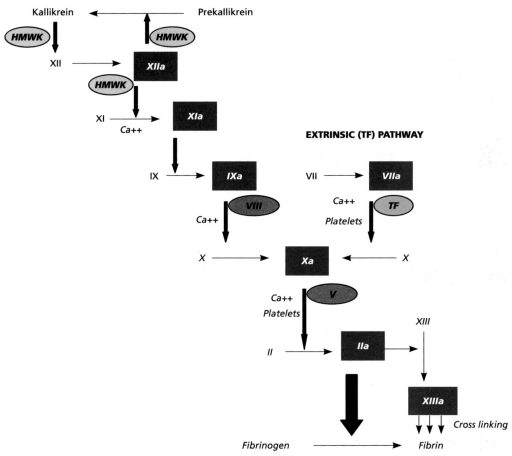

EXTRINSIC (TF) PATHWAY

Figure 18.2 Blood coagulation is now seen as a network of interactions triggered by contact of blood with extravascular tissue factor (TF). The initial conversion of factor X to Xa by the TF-VIIa leads to generation of small quantities of thrombin (IIa) which back-activate V and VIII. Rapid thrombin generation then proceeds with feedback to FXI and converts soluble fibrinogen to insoluble fibrin. The intrinsic pathway is less important as an initiator of blood coagulation in higher animals. (HMWK; high molecular weight kininogen)

Q13 What other possibility could explain the abnormal coagulation screen in the baby?

A Vitamin K deficiency results in impaired synthesis of factors II, VII, IX and X, and proteins C and S, and may cause haemorrhagic disease in newborn infants. This is unlikely here as the PT is normal and both the PT and APTT would be prolonged with vitamin K deficiency.

Q14 What should be done if vitamin K deficiency is suspected?

A Vitamin K should be given intravenously.

> **Key point**
> Vitamin K should not be given intramuscularly as the baby obviously has a bleeding defect and this could cause a deep haematoma (bleeding into a muscle).

Q15 What should the mother be told at this stage?

A It is likely that the baby has a congenital bleeding disorder. A specific diagnosis should be available within 24–48 hours. Most congenital bleeding disorders can be easily treated.

Q16 What further blood tests should be ordered?

A Measurement of the factor VIII and factor IX levels in the baby's blood.

Factor VIII and factor IX deficiency are the commonest inherited bleeding disorders that present with bleeding in the neonatal period. Factor VIII deficiency is 6 times more common than factor IX deficiency. The result of factor VIII and factor IX assays are shown in Table 18.4.

Table 18.4 Factor VIII and IX assays

	Patient's result	Normal range
Factor VIII	0%	22–139%
Factor IX	64%	10–66%

A Factor VIII is absent in the baby's plasma. This is compatible with a diagnosis of severe haemophilia A.

Key point

Haemophilia is caused by mutations of the FVIII gene (haemophilia A) or FIX gene (haemophilia B) on the X chromosome. Approximately 1 male child out of 5000 is affected by haemophilia A. Over 200 mutations in the large and complex FVIII gene lead to inadequate synthesis of FVIII and hence thrombin generation is impaired. Approximately 50% of all haemophilia A is due to an inversion of intron 22, which simplifies the diagnosis and genetic counselling.

Q18 Why is the gender of the child important?

A The gene for factor VIII is present on the X chromosome and this disease is, therefore, called an 'X-linked disease'. This means that the disease manifests itself in boys but that girls can be 'carriers' (Fig. 18.3).

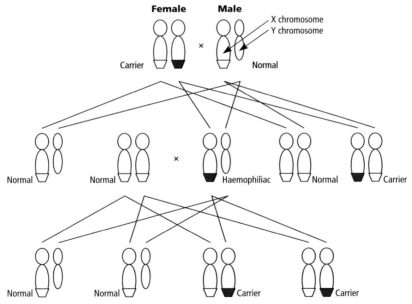

Figure 18.3 X-linked inheritance. Three chromosomes are shown, a normal X (tip of long arm unshaded), an X bearing a mutant factor VIII gene (tip of long arm shaded) and a normal Y. A female carrier with a normal partner has four types of offspring with equal frequency: normal son, haemophiliac son, normal daughter and carrier daughter. A haemophiliac male with a normal partner has only two types of offspring: carrier daughters and normal sons.

A About 30 to 50% of children with haemophilia have no family history of abnormal bleeding. This is due to spontaneous mutations in the factor VIII or IX gene.

Q20 What level of factor VIII is present in carriers (girls who pass on haemophilia to their children)?

A The levels of factor VIII in carriers are variable because of random X chromosome inactivation known as 'Lyonization' (Fig. 18.4).

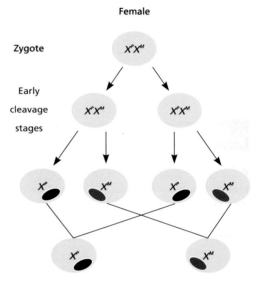

Figure 18.4 Lyonization (after Mary Lyon) is the name given to the process of inactivation of one member of the pair of X chromosomes in every female cell. It occurs in all somatic cells of the female embryo on the 16th day after fertilization when the embryo comprises around 5000 cells. For any somatic cell, the choice as to whether the paternal (X^P) or the maternal (X^M) X chromosome is inactivated is random (the inactive X is shown as a dark mass). Hence, normal females are mosaics with a mixture of X^M and X^P. Because of the intrinsic randomness of the inactivation process, the relative proportions of gene-protein expression vary from female to female. This accounts for the variable expression of X-linked recessive traits in heterozygous females, who may be symptomatic if most cells are utilizing the defective gene on the X chromosome.

A The mother should be told that factor VIII replacement therapy will stop the bleeding and with appropriate treatment her child should have a normal life expectancy.

> **Key point**
> Bleeding must be treated promptly and appropriately. The dose of FVIII replacement is determined by its volume of distribution, the half-life, and the haemostatic requirement of the type of bleeding. Haemarthroses and soft tissue bleeds require 30–40% correction, while life-threatening haemorrhages require 80–100%. Prophylactic use of concentrates, which prevent severe bleeding, is now commonly recommended.

Q22 From where is factor VIII concentrate derived?

A Factor VIII concentrates are made from human plasma or from genetically engineered mammalian cells.

Q23 What risks does the administration of a concentrate from human plasma carry?

A The administration of blood products made from human plasma always carries the potential risk of transmitting viral or other infections. However, the combination of strict donor viral screening protocols and intensive donor self-exclusion programmes together with viral inactivation processes have prevented HIV or hepatitis C transmission from the use of plasma-derived factor concentrates since the late 1980s. These viral inactivation steps are not effective against parvovirus B19, hepatitis A or Creutzfeld–Jakob prions.

> **Key point**
> Recombinant coagulation factor products offer the best possible protection from transmission of human blood-borne viruses and are regarded as the treatment of choice for all patients with haemophilia.

A Yes.

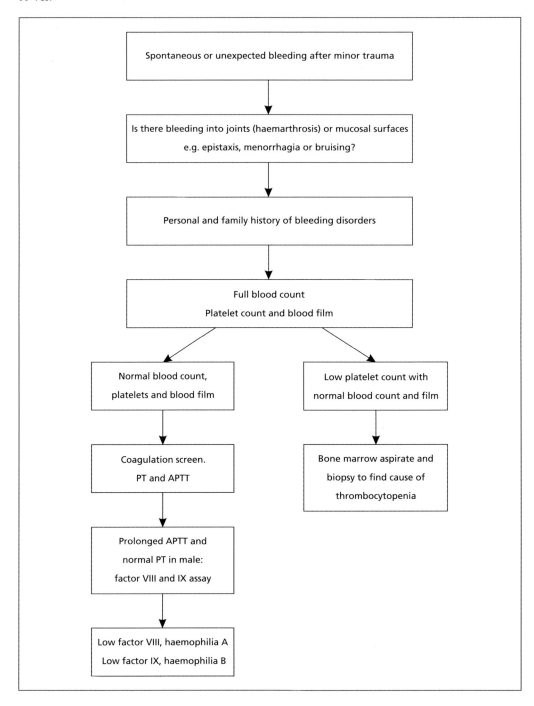

OUTCOME

The baby was treated with recombinant FVIII (25 U/kg) intravenously twice daily for 3 days. Cranial ultrasound showed no evidence of intraventricular haemorrhage. The child was subsequently referred to a paediatric hae-mophilia centre, where he attended every 3 months. At the age of 18 months prophylactic replacement therapy was commenced because he had sustained numerous bleeds into his knee joint.

Suggested reading

Michele, D. (1996) Hemophilia 1996: new approach to an old disease. *Pediatric Clinics of North America*, **43** (3), 709–36.

Colman, R.W., Hirsh, J., Marder, V.J., Clowes, A.W. & George, J.N. (2001) *Haemostasis and Thrombosis: Basic Principles & Clinical Practice*, 4th edn. Lippincott Williams & Wilkins, Hagerstown, USA.

Kitchens, C.S., Alving, B.M. & Kessler, C.M. (eds) (2002) *Consultative Haemostasis and Thrombosis*. W.B. Saunders Company, Philadelphia, USA.

Smith, O.P. & Hann I.M. (eds) (2002) *Essential Paediatric Haematology*. Martin Dunitz, London, UK.

World Federation of Haemophilia: www.wfh.com

A young lady with chest pain following a long plane journey

Six hours following her return from Australia to Ireland, Jane, a 26-year-old pharmacist, developed chest pain. The chest pain was predominantly down her left side and because it was so severe she requested her general practitioner (GP) to come to her home.

Q1 What should the doctor do?

A Arrange to take her to the nearest Accident and Emergency (A&E) department.

Q2 What should be done on arrival at the A&E department?

A A full history and physical examination should be carried out.

Q3 What aspects of the history should the doctor in the A&E department concentrate on?

A A history of any previous similar episode or leg swelling. A family history of similar complaints.

Physical examination was unremarkable apart from the reduced air entry in her left lung and that her chest pain was made worse by deep inspiration. She was hypoxaemic (O_2 saturation 90% on room air; normal >96%).

Q4 What is the most likely diagnosis from what you know so far?

A Pulmonary embolism (PE). A large spontaneous pneumothorax could present in the same way.

Q5 What should be done next?

A A chest radiograph, coagulation screen (Table 19.1) and an electrocardiograph (ECG).

The chest radiograph was normal and the ECG showed a sinus tachycardia.

Table 19.1 Coagulation screen

Tests	Patient's results	Normal range
Prothrombin time, PT	13 sec	12–15 sec
Activated partial thromboplastin time, APTT	40 sec	25–35 sec

Q6 How do the chest radiographic findings, ECG and coagulation results help to confirm your suspicion of a PE?

A Neither the ECG nor the chest radiograph point to a specific diagnosis and the coagulation screen is normal.

Q7 What further test should be done to make the diagnosis?

A Ventilation perfusions scan of the lungs (Figs 19.1 and 19.2).

The V/Q scan indicates bilateral perfusion defects consistent with an embolus in the pulmonary circulation (PE).

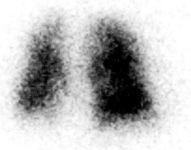

Figure 19.1 A xenon ventilation scan showing a normal lung pattern.

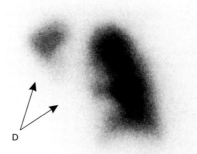

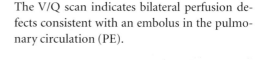

Figure 19.2 ^{99m}Tc MAA perfusion scan demonstrating multiple perfusion defects (D), particularly in the left lung. Multiple perfusion defects with a normal radiograph and ventilation scan makes a PE the likely diagnosis.

Q8 What should be done next?

A The patient should be given oxygen support, adequate pain relief and anticoagulation with heparin.

Heparin is available in unfractionated or low molecular weight forms (LMWH).

 Q9 How can a normal coagulation screen be reconciled with a PE in an otherwise healthy young patient?

A Inherited prothrombotic states (thrombophilia) may dispose to venous thrombosis/emboli with a normal coagulation screen.

Q10 What further blood test will help to confirm if an embolus has occurred?

A D-dimer measurement (Table 19.2).

Table 19.2 Results of D-dimer test

	Patient's result	Normal value
D-dimer	6000 µg/ml	<200 µg/ml

Q11 How can the elevated D-dimers be explained?

A D-dimers are elevated in the plasma following the conversion of fibrinogen to fibrin during clot formation and the subsequent breakdown of fibrin by plasmin.

Q12 How could the family history help to determine if Jane has a prothrombotic state?

A It is common to find a history of embolism in first-degree relatives.

> **Key point**
> Many prothrombotic states are inherited and often due to single mutations of proteins in the anticoagulant pathway.

A Smoking, oral contraceptives and ethnic background (Fig. 19.3).

Women of child-bearing age should also be asked about a history of recurrent spontaneous abortion, intrauterine growth retardation and pre-eclampsia.

Jane had been taking oral contraceptives for 3 years and two of her first cousins developed clots in their leg veins during and after pregnancy.

Key point

Venous thrombosis/emboli (VTE) which occur following long haul air flights have been given the name 'economy class syndrome'. This results from sitting in a cramped position without adequate exercise and probable dehydration accentuated by alcohol ingestion. The majority of patients, however, who have the 'economy class syndrome' have risk factors for venous thrombosis.

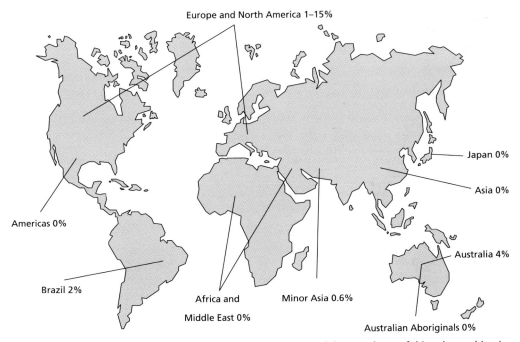

Figure 19.3 The factor V Leiden allele is found only in Caucasians and the prevalence of this polymorphism in the general population of Western societies has considerable variation. High prevalence (up to 15%) is found in southern Sweden, in Germany, Greece and Israel. In the Netherlands, UK, Ireland and the USA, around 3–5% of the population carry the mutant alleles. Lower prevalence, around 2%, is found in Hispanics.

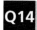 **Q14** How might you investigate what types of inherited coagulation disorder can give rise to prothrombotic states?

A Look for inherited deficiencies of protein C, protein S and polymorphisms of factor V or prothrombin. These inherited deficiencies can be measured by more sophisticated clotting assays or by genetic tests (Table 19.3).

Further investigation revealed factor V Leiden (the commonest coagulation factor variant leading to a prothrombotic state). These inherited abnormalities are called thrombophilia.

Table 19.3 Inherited thrombophilia

Type of abnormality	Investigations
Protein C deficiency	Clotting test
Protein S deficiency	Clotting test
Factor V Leiden	Clotting test and genetic test
Prothrombin G202 10A	Genetic test

 Q15 What advantage does low molecular weight heparin have over unfractionated heparin when treating Jane?

A Low molecular weight heparin has a long plasma half-life and a more predictable dose response, making monitoring with blood tests unnecessary other than in pregnancy and renal failure.

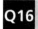 **Q16** For how long should anticoagulation be continued after initial heparinization?

A The anticoagulant warfarin can be started within 24 hours of the heparin treatment and should be continued for 6 months.

> **Key point**
> Women with thrombophilia who use the oral contraceptive pill (OCP) develop blood clots more often and sooner after initiation of the OCP than women without thrombophilia.

Q17 How would you consider carrying out population studies to detect inherited thrombophilia?

A It is practical only in young women with a family history of thromboses or known thrombophilia.

Q18 What method of contraception should Jane be advised to use?

A Barrier methods or medroxyprogesterone (a depo injection every 3 months).

Q19 What advice should be given to people with inherited thrombophilia before undertaking long flights or journeys?

A They should be advised to wear support stockings, exercise hourly and refrain from alcohol.

Q20 What drug could be used as a prophylaxis against VTE in these individuals?

A Low molecular weight heparin given shortly before the flight.

> **Key point**
> Aspirin has been recommended but would be totally ineffectual in preventing VTE and may cause gastric irritation and bleeding (see Case 17).

Can you now construct an algorithm for a young woman with sudden onset of severe chest pain?

A Yes.

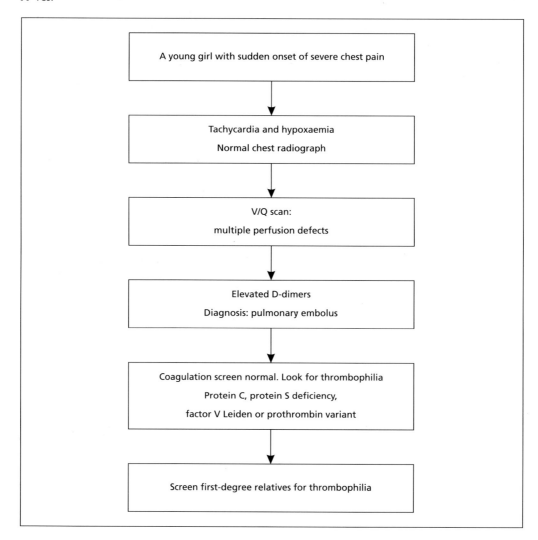

A young girl with sudden onset of severe chest pain

↓

Tachycardia and hypoxaemia

Normal chest radiograph

↓

V/Q scan:

multiple perfusion defects

↓

Elevated D-dimers

Diagnosis: pulmonary embolus

↓

Coagulation screen normal. Look for thrombophilia

Protein C, protein S deficiency,

factor V Leiden or prothrombin variant

↓

Screen first-degree relatives for thrombophilia

OUTCOME

Jane was commenced on LMWH at therapeutic doses without monitoring. She was sent home the next day after commencing warfarin with daily monitoring. She was treated for 6 months in total. A year later, Jane became pregnant and was given prophylactic LMWH. Her pregnancy was uneventful. Given her history of VTE and FV Leiden, prophylactic LMWH was administered throughout her pregnancy and for a further 6 weeks postpartum with no recurrence of thrombotic episodes. Both of her cousins were heterozygous for the FV Leiden polymorphism.

Suggested reading

Bauer, K.A. (1995) Management of patients with hereditary defects predisposing to thrombosis including pregnant women. *Thrombosis and Haemostasis*, **74**, 94–100.

Colman, R.W., Hirsh, J., Marder, V.J., Clowes, A.W. & George, J.N. (eds) (2001) *Haemostasis and Thrombosis: Basic Principles & Clinical Practice*, 4th edn. Lippincott Williams & Wilkins, Hagerstown, USA.

Goodnight, S.H., Jr & Hathaway, W.E. (2001) *Disorders of Hemostasis & Thrombosis: A Clinical Guide*, 2nd edn. McGraw Hill, New York, USA.

Kitchens, C.S., Alving, B.M. & Kessler, C.M. (eds) (2002) *Consultative Haemostasis and Thrombosis*. W.B. Saunders & Company, St Louis, USA.

Khoury, M.J., McCabe, L.L. & McCabe, E.R.B. (2003) Population screening in the age of genomic medicine. *New England Journal of Medicine*, **348** (1), 50–8.

CASE 20

'Doctor, will I get an infection from the blood transfusion?'

Catherine, a 27-year-old schoolteacher, was involved in a motorcar accident. She was taken to the nearest Accident and Emergency department, where she was given emergency care and transferred to the orthopaedic department. She had a fractured pelvis and right tibia and a laceration on her face, which required suturing.

She had never been in hospital before. She was not taking any medications. She is married but has no children. She is a non-smoker and non-drinker.

Investigations revealed the following (Table 20.1). The blood film showed polychromasia (Fig. 20.1).

Table 20.1 Full blood count

	Patient's results	Normal range
Hb	7.9 g/dl	11.5–16.4 g/dl
MCV	96 fl	83.0–99.0 fl (µm^3)
WBC	12.0 × 10^9/l	4.0–11.0 × 10^9/l (10^3/µl)
Neutrophils	10.0 × 10^9/l	2.0–7.5 × 10^9/l (10^3/µl)
Lymphocytes	2.0 × 10^9/l	1.5–3.5 × 10^9/l (10^3/µl)
Platelets	500 × 10^9/l	140–450 × 10^9/l (10^3/µl)

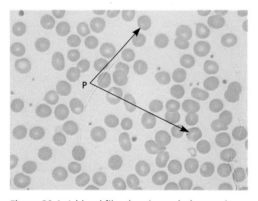

Figure 20.1 A blood film showing polychromasia (P).

Q1 What is the explanation for the blood findings?

A The anaemia is probably caused by blood loss following the fractures. The polychromasia reflects an increased number of reticulocytes. The word 'polychromasia' refers to the blue/grey colour of these cells, which reflects the ribosomal content. The slightly raised neutrophil and platelet count are a response to the bleeding. A large number of platelets are normally present in the spleen. Following major trauma they are released into the circulation, accounting for the rise in the platelet count.

Q2 How should this patient be managed?

A The facial laceration should be sutured immediately.

She will require a general anaesthetic and surgery to reduce the fracture of her tibia. The pelvic fracture is stable and does not require surgery.

Q3 Why might she require blood transfusion?

A Her Hb is <8.0 g/dl and she is actively bleeding. There may be more blood loss at the time of surgery. A rapid onset of anaemia, such as happened here following the accident, may lead to hypovolemic 'shock' and should be treated with blood transfusion.

Although there is no absolute Hb level at which blood transfusion is indicated, a 'transfusion trigger' of 8.0 g/dl is commonly taken as an indication for blood transfusion. A decision to recommend blood transfusion will depend on the cause and speed of onset of the anaemia as well as the patient's age and general health. Anaemia which is gradual in onset is often well tolerated by the patient and if the underlying cause is corrected a blood transfusion may not be necessary.

Q4 Before requesting blood for this patient what further information is required?

A A past history of blood transfusion and pregnancies (whether they ended prematurely, naturally or by abortion) is essential.

A Antibodies may be formed to antigens on the transfused or foetal red cells.

Red blood cells have a number of antigens, which are expressed on the cell surface. During blood transfusion not all of these antigens are identified (especially the rare ones). If a patient receives red cells with antigens that are different from the antigens on the patient's own red cells, he or she may make antibodies to these foreign antigens. These antibodies may not cause a problem and may be present in small amounts in the patient's blood. If, at a future date, another blood transfusion is given with the same foreign antigens on the red cells, a 'haemolytic' transfusion reaction may take place where the antibodies in the patient's blood attack the transfused red blood cells. This can result in destruction of all the transfused cells and renal failure. It can be fatal.

> **Key point**
>
> At the time of delivery or abortion, red cells from the foetus may cross into the mother's circulation. The mother may make antibodies (foetal red cells have antigens from both parents). As in Q5, future blood transfusions may cause similar problems.

A Antibodies can cross the placenta from the mother and cause haemolysis in the foetus.

A rhesus negative mother who has a rhesus positive baby may develop antibodies. These antibodies may increase in amount in the mother's circulation in subsequent pregnancies and cross the placenta (this time in the opposite direction) from the mother to the foetus and cause destruction of the foetal red cells.

When it is established that the patient never had a pregnancy or blood transfusion, the necessity for a transfusion should be explained.

A It is safer to have a blood transfusion than risk further anaemia from the blood loss.

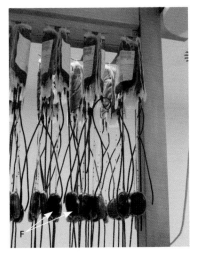

Figure 20.2 White cells being removed by filtration (F) from whole blood.

Key point

Transfusion of any blood product will always carry the risk of transmitting an infectious agent.

Previously, transmission of the human immunodeficiency virus (HIV) via blood and blood products (especially clotting factor concentrates) resulted in a human tragedy, with illness and death for many patients. Transmission occurred **before** the virus had been identified. Blood and blood products transmitted hepatitis C virus, again **before** the virus had been identified. Malaria can also be transmitted, and more recently West Nile virus has been transmitted by blood transfusion.

To minimize the possibility of prion transmission (vCJd) and to reduce the number of febrile transfusion reactions, white cells can be removed from red cells after collection (Fig. 20.2).

Q8 What has changed in the world of blood transfusion to make blood and blood products safer?

A Careful screening of blood donors, and treatment of blood to remove infectious agents.

1 Careful screening of all blood donors, including a detailed history and a number of intrusive questions about sexual history, travel and substance abuse (Table 20.2).
2 Screening the blood of donors for antibodies, and more recently nucleic acid sequences, from the 'known' viruses.
3 Viral inactivation of blood products. This does not apply to red blood cell transfusions.

4 A widespread public campaign making people aware of the dangers of donating if they are possibly infected with one of the viruses mentioned.
5 Not allowing volunteers to donate blood until the incubation period has passed if they have visited an area where a particular virus is causing infection (e.g. parts of the USA for West Nile virus).
6 Making sure that new donors are screened on two occasions before blood is taken for transfusion.

Table 20.2 Questions asked of a potential donor

1 Are you giving blood to be tested for HIV/AIDS or hepatitis?
2 Have you ever injected or been injected with non-prescription drugs – even once or a long time ago? This includes bodybuilding drugs.
3 If you are a male, have you ever had oral or anal sex with another male – even if a condom or other protective was used?
4 Have you ever received money or drugs for sex?
5 Do you or your partner have HIV/AIDS?
6 Do you or your partner or close household contacts have hepatitis B or C?
If the answer to any of the above is YES, or if you are in any doubt, you must indicate YES, and NOT donate.

From the Irish Blood Transfusion Service Donor Health Questionnaire

Q9 What is meant by the term 'blood products'?

A Blood contains cells (red cells, white cells and platelets) and liquid (plasma) in which proteins and clotting factors are present (Table 20.3).

Table 20.3 Blood products

Packed red cells	When blood is collected from a donor it is centrifuged, the white cells are removed by filtration, and the platelets and plasma are saved for further use (Fig. 20.3). The red cells are suspended in a preservative solution and can be used for up to 35 days. Packed red cells **cannot** be treated to inactivate viruses.
Platelets	Platelets for transfusion may be separated from blood at the time of collection and suspended in plasma until they are ready for use (up to 5 days). Alternatively, the donor may be attached to a machine where blood is continuously centrifuged and a large number of platelets removed and stored for transfusion (Fig. 20.4). The red blood cells and plasma are returned to the donor. This is called platelet pheresis and is equivalent to individual collections from five donors. Platelets **cannot** be treated to inactivate viruses.
Plasma	Plasma can be collected from individual units of blood (Fig. 20.5) or collected by plasma pheresis. Plasma can be frozen and stored for 2 years before use. Plasma **can** be treated to inactivate viruses.
Factor 'concentrates'	Factors VIII, IX, VII and fibrinogen can be made into 'concentrates' for replacement therapy (Fig. 20.6). Plasma is 'pooled' from many donors. All these 'concentrates' **can** be treated to inactivate viruses. Because of the possibility of transmitting viral infections, so-called 'recombinant' products are also available. These recombinant products are manufactured by transfecting animal 'cell lines' with the human gene for the particular factor required, e.g. factor VIII gene into Chinese hamster ovary cells. These products are frozen and need to be reconstituted before use.

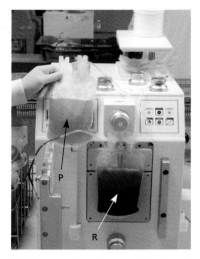

Figure 20.3 Preparation of red cells for transfusion. Plasma is removed and red cells (R) suspended in a preservative solution.

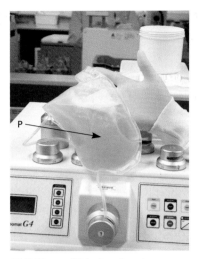

Figure 20.5 Plasma (P) before freezing.

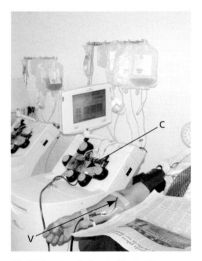

Figure 20.4 Platelets being collected by centrifugation, showing cannula from the donor's vein (V) to the continuous-flow centrifuge (C).

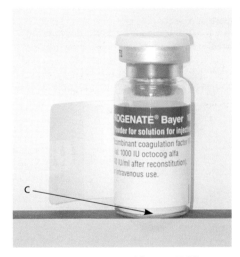

Figure 20.6 A concentrate of factor VIII (C).

Q10 How has the introduction of these measures made a difference in terms of safety of blood transfusion?

A The public campaign, screening of donors and measures to remove infectious agents has reduced the risk of transmitting disease by blood transfusion.

> ### Key point
> The risk of transmitting known viruses is now so low that it cannot be quantified and must be estimated using mathematical models (Table 20.4).

Many individuals 'screened' themselves out of the donor pool when they realized that gay men were possibly transmitting human immunodeficiency virus (HIV) via blood **before** the test to detect antibodies to HIV was introduced.

Table 20.4 Estimated frequency of transmitting viral infections by blood

Hepatitis B*	1 in 250 000
HIV	1 in 8 million
Hepatitis C virus, HCV	1 in 30 million

*Although the estimate is 1 in 250 000, the actual incidence seems to be much lower and with widespread use of new tests will be significantly less than 1 in 250 000.

Q11 What is meant by a 'window period'?

A A 'lag' period after a viral infection, before antibodies are produced in the infected individual.

> ### Key point
> If the Transfusion Service is testing donors for antibodies, it is possible that an infected donor could be 'missed' as the donation might be taken after a viral infection and before the antibodies can be detected. The introduction of nucleic acid sequence testing will detect the virus immediately after infection.

Q12 What other precautions are taken prior to blood transfusion?

A The blood sample is examined for the antigens present on the red blood cells (blood group) and carefully labelled before it is transferred to the hospital for use. Usually, a bar code (similar to the supermarket type) is used to check the identity of the patient and the blood for donation.

A sample of blood from the patient is examined to determine the blood group, and the patient's blood is examined for the presence of blood group antibodies that might be present from a previous transfusion or pregnancy.

A Human error.

The most common cause of a blood transfusion problem is failure to identify the patient and the donated blood correctly due to a human mistake (misreading the label, giving the wrong blood and providing the wrong patient information on the request form).

Q14 Can you construct an algorithm for safe blood transfusion?

A Yes.

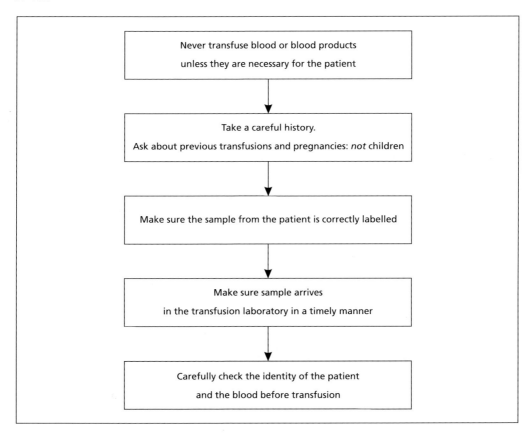

Never transfuse blood or blood products
unless they are necessary for the patient

↓

Take a careful history.
Ask about previous transfusions and pregnancies: *not* children

↓

Make sure the sample from the patient is correctly labelled

↓

Make sure sample arrives
in the transfusion laboratory in a timely manner

↓

Carefully check the identity of the patient
and the blood before transfusion

OUTCOME

Catherine received 3 units of blood and had her surgery safely. She was advised to take iron tablets for 3 months. She was discharged from hospital 3 weeks later and attended the physiotherapy department until she had fully recovered. Two years later she had a normal healthy baby.

Key point

Over 50% of patients who receive a blood transfusion die within 2 years of their underlying disease. This statistic, however, does not apply to neonates, pregnant women and many trauma victims.

Some religious beliefs forbid the use of blood transfusion (e.g. Jehovah's Witnesses). With careful management, diseases such as leukaemia have been successfully treated without the use of blood transfusions.

Suggested reading

Mintz, P.D. (1999) *Transfusion Therapy: Clinical Principles and Practice,* AABB Press, Belhesda, USA.

Hoffbrand, A.V., Pettit, J.E. & Moss, P.A.H. (2001) *Essential Haematology,* 4th edn. Blackwell Science, Oxford. See Chapter 23: Blood transfusion.

Mazza, P., Prudenzano, A., Amurri, B. *et al.* (2003) Myeloablative therapy and bone marrow transplantation in Jehovah's Witnesses with malignancies: single centre experience. *Bone Marrow Transplantation,* 32, 433–6.

Prowse, C.V. (2003) An ABC for West Nile virus. *Transfusion Medicine,* 13, 1–7.

Soldan, K., Barbara, J.A.J., Ramsay, M.E. & Hall, A.J. (2003) Estimation of the risk of hepatitis B virus, hepatitis C virus and human immunodeficiency virus infectious donations entering the blood supply in England, 1993–2001. *Vox Sanguinis,* 84, 274–86.

Index

West Nile virus 169
white cell count (WBC), elevated **80,** 81, 86, 90

white cells
  precursors 81
  removal from whole blood 169

X chromosome inactivation *154*
X-linked inheritance 153